Diagnosis and Treatment of Common Skin Diseases

K. Bork

and

W. Bräuninger

Dermatology Clinic
University of Mainz
Mainz, West Germany

Translated from the Original German Text by
Karl H. Mueller, M.D.
and
Hendrik K. Mueller

Adapted by Carla A. Skibba, M.D.

The Medical College of Wisconsin
Milwaukee, Wisconsin

Diagnosis and Treatment of Common Skin Diseases

W.B. SAUNDERS COMPANY
Harcourt Brace Jovanovich, Inc.
Philadelphia London Toronto Montreal Sydney Tokyo

W. B. SAUNDERS COMPANY
Harcourt Brace Jovanovich, Inc.

The Curtis Center
Independence Square West
Philadelphia, PA 19106

Library of Congress Cataloging-in-Publication Data

Bork, K. (Konrad)

Diagnosis and treatment of common skin diseases.

Translation of: Erkennung und Behandlung haufiger
Hautkrankheiten.

1. Skin—Diseases.   I. Bräuninger, W.   II. Title.
   [DNLM: 1. Skin Diseases—diagnosis.   2. Skin Diseases—
   therapy. WR 140 B734e]

RL71.B67713   1988   616.5   88–15645

ISBN 0–7216–2240–2

Translators' Note

   Recommendations for therapy throughout this book are based on the experience of the authors and their colleagues at the dermatology clinic of the University Hospital, Mainz. Where possible the names of German therapeutic preparations have been replaced in this English edition by equivalent United States product names. Some German products have no exact United States equivalent or must be compounded, and these are designated by appropriate notes in the text, particularly in the final chapter on therapy. Treatment methods described are not necessarily those that would be recommended by the translators.

Editor: Albert Meier
Cover Artist: Ellen Bodner
Production Manager: Carolyn Naylor
Manuscript Editor: Patrice Smith
Indexer: George Vilk

Authorized English edition of ERKENNUNG UND BEHANDLUNG HAUFIGER HAUTKRANKHEITEN, © 1986 by F.K. Schattauer Verlag, Stuttgart.

Diagnosis and Treatment of Common Skin Diseases   ISBN 0–7216–2240–2

Last digit is the print number: 9   8   7   6   5   4

Preface

The physician in private practice sees a great number of dermatologic problems and must constantly review and update his or her knowledge of diagnostic criteria and current therapy. This book was written to assist in this task. We have tried to give a synopsis of clinical aspects and treatment of common dermatoses with special emphasis on pictorial presentation of the typical symptoms and signs and their most frequent variants. Rare skin diseases, as well as theoretic discussions of pathogenesis and histology, literature references, and so on were omitted to make the book more useful for the practitioner. Differential diagnostic criteria were included only where they were absolutely necessary. Therapeutic measures found to be effective and useful in practice are discussed in detail. Treatment methods requiring hospitalization of the patient were mentioned where indicated but were not described further.

This book was written for the primary care physician and should also be useful for internists and pediatricians.

In the German edition the diseases are presented in alphabetical order, but this could not be done in the American edition without reorganizing both the text and the color plates.

We are indebted to Prof. Dr. med. Dr. H. C. P. Matis and the Schattauer Publishing Company who so generously accepted our suggestions regarding the publication of this book and especially the many color illustrations. We owe a special debt of gratitude to Prof. Dr. G. W. Korting, Director of the Dermatology Clinic of the University of Mainz, for his support. We thank Prof. Dr. W. Stille, Center for Internal Medicine of the University of Frankfurt, for Figures 305 to 307 and Prof. Dr. G. K. Steigleder, Director of the Dermatology Clinic, University of Cologne, for Figure 308. We also wish to express our gratitude to Mr. G. Faber, the photographer for our clinic, and to Miss E. Lennartz, our devoted secretary, for their excellent work.

K. BORK, W. BRÄUNINGER

Contents

Diagnosis and Treatment of Common Skin Diseases

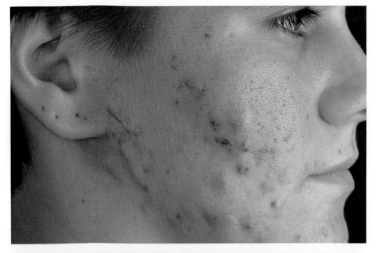

Figure 1. Acne vulgaris. Solitary comedos, inflammatory nodules, and isolated pustules on the right cheek. The enlarged follicle openings are clearly visible.

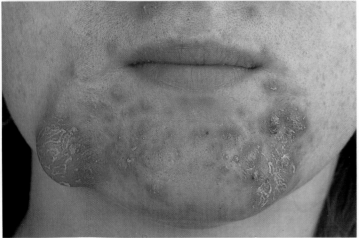

Figure 2. Nodular and cystic acne vulgaris, involving mainly the chin area ("chin acne").

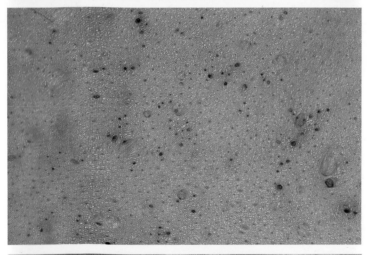

Figure 3. Acne vulgaris with multiple comedos and small residual scars.

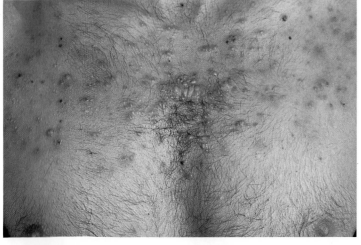

Figure 4. Acne vulgaris. Multiple pustules and keloid formation as they are frequently found on the chest.

Part I

Common Skin Diseases

Acne

Acne vulgaris is one of the most common skin disorders seen by the practicing physician. It occurs during puberty in approximately 75 percent of all adolescents but varies in severity. The disorder rarely lasts longer than 10 years and usually disappears in early adulthood. Severe nodular or nodular-cystic involvement is found mainly in young men. In women 20 to 35 years of age, nodules are frequently found in the perioral area or on the chin (chin acne). Inflammatory lesions can lead to disfiguring scar formation, which makes competent treatment of acne an important task for the attending physician. It is not just "cosmetic therapy." Heredity plays a significant etiologic role, as well as a number of other factors, such as excessive production of sebum (seborrhea), with the formation of free fatty acids, bacterial contamination of the follicles of sebaceous glands with Propionibacterium acnes, *stimulation of sebum production by androgens, and altered keratinization of the follicular infundibulum. Psychologic factors may also play a role and must be treated appropriately.*

Acne Vulgaris

Clinical Appearance

Acne presents with a colorful variety of efflorescences.

1. The primary lesion is a comedo without inflammatory changes (blackhead) whose dark discoloration is caused by melanin. Secondary inflammation of the follicular apparatus leads to formation of erythematous papules, papulopustular lesions, and pustules. In more severe cases, nodules and abscesses with fistulae can develop, often aggravated by the patient's own manipulations. This frequently results in severe scar formation, especially when therapy is inadequate.
2. Acne is located primarily in the face; the chest and upper back may also be involved.
3. There is generalized seborrhea with oily facial skin and a disposition for greasy hair.

Therapy

Treatment is symptomatic and must be continued as long as comedones and inflammation are present, usually over a period of several years.

External

1. In order to remove the grease, the skin should be cleansed with a mild soap.
2. Benzoyl peroxide is very effective against papular and pustular lesions. The base of the medication must be chosen according to the condition of the skin (alcohol gel for very oily skin [R.24a], watery gel for less oily skin [R.24a], and emulsions for sensitive skin, especially of the face [R.42a]).
3. Tretinoin (vitamin A acid) solutions are more effective than gels (R.24b) or creams (R.42b) but can more easily lead to irritation of the skin. Tretinoin-containing preparations are effective against comedones, less effective against papular and pustular lesions.
4. Removal of unacceptable comedones must be performed by a competent technician. Excessive pressing and squeezing should be avoided.
5. Incision of cysts and purulent nodules should be performed only by a physician.
6. Intralesional injection of a corticosteroid crystal suspension into the larger nodular lesions can occasionally be helpful.
7. Cosmetically unacceptable scars can be treated by dermabrasion, after the inflammatory changes have subsided. It is desirable, however, to prevent such scar formation by early competent therapy of acne lesions.

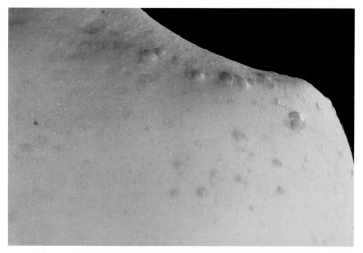

Figure 5. Acne vulgaris. Scars and keloids on the right shoulder.

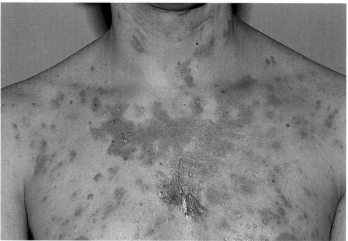

Figure 6. Acne conglobata. Deep folliculitis and extensive fresh scarring with beginning keloid formation on the chest.

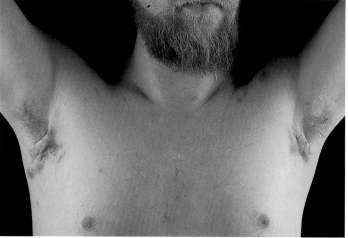

Figure 7. Chronic abscess formation with extensive scarring in both axillae in a patient with acne conglobata.

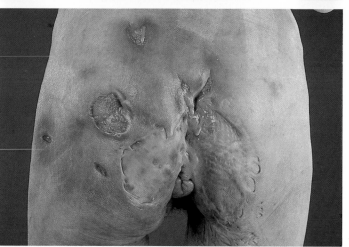

Figure 8. Acne conglobata. Severe involvement of many years' duration with recurrent development of nodules, abscesses, and fistulae, as well as extensive scarring in the perianal and gluteal areas. Appearance after repeated operative procedures and skin grafts.

1. The role of diet in the treatment of acne is often emphasized in the lay press, but there is no evidence to support its effectiveness. Many acne patients are already psychologically influenced by their disease and should not be burdened with a useless diet.

2. Female patients may benefit from a supplemental therapy with antiandrogens in combination with estrogens. (Diane, or cyproteronacetate, as recommended by the original German text, is also an effective oral contraceptive. It contains cyproterone acetate 2 mg and ethinyl estradiol 0.5 mg.) Compared with this regimen, other oral contraceptives are less effective, if at all. The beneficial effect of systemic corticosteroids is at least questionable. Long-term therapy may even worsen acne.

3. Systemic antibiotics (tetracyclines [R.47] or erythromycin [R.49]) are useful in the treatment of inflammatory acne. We begin with 1 gm per day of the antibiotic until significant improvement has been achieved. Treatment is then continued for several months with a lower maintenance dose (usually 250 mg per day). The influence of this treatment on the intestinal flora is minimal.

Acne Conglobata

It is practical to discuss this severe form of acne separately from acne vulgaris. Acne conglobata occurs more frequently in men; its course is usually prolonged.

Clinical Appearance

1. The comedo is the primary lesion, as in acne vulgaris. Additionally, there are conglomerates of comedones and giant comedones. Inflammatory changes with the formation of abscesses and fistulae are more extensive than in acne vulgaris.

2. In addition to the sites usually affected by acne vulgaris, acne conglobata can also involve the entire trunk, the arms, and the neck. In severe cases, the axillae, groin, and perianal region can also be involved (acne triade; acne tetrade).

3. Patients with acne conglobata frequently have a distinct tendency for the formation of keloid scars and severe seborrhea.

Therapy

External

Topical treatment is the same as that for acne vulgaris (see earlier).

Systemic

Isotretinoin (a derivative of vitamin A) is the treatment of choice for acne conglobata (R.60). The daily dose is 0.5 to 1 mg per kg body weight per day and is given in treatment cycles of 16 weeks.

Surgical procedures are occasionally necessary for the treatment of chronic fistulae or extensive scars with restriction of motion, especially in the axilla. Systemic medical treatment of the disease, however, takes precedence.

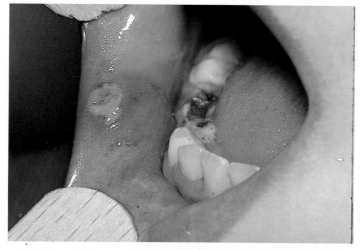

Figure 9. Recurrent aphthae. Fresh aphtha with yellow fibrin coating and erythematous border.

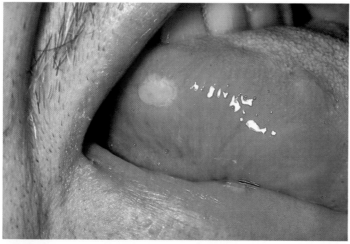

Figure 10. Recurrent aphthae. Aphtha of the tongue with adherent fibrinous coating.

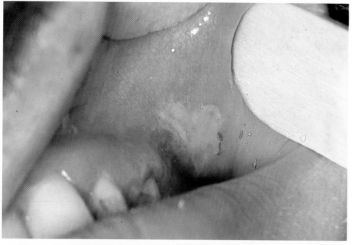

Figure 11. Recurrent aphthae. Large fresh aphtha with curvilinear border in the upper mucobuccal fold.

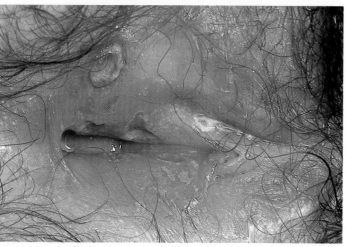

Figure 12. Recurrent aphthae. Deep genital aphthae of the labia minora and majora.

Aphthae

Recurrent Aphthae

Recurrent aphthae are painful erosions or ulcers of the mucous membrane of the mouth that usually last for several days. Their etiology is not known, but immunologic mechanisms seem to play a role in their pathogenesis. Certain foods (nuts, chocolate, tomatoes) can occasionally cause an acute attack. It is important to distinguish recurrent aphthae from other diseases with aphthoid stomatitis, such as drug reactions, infections with enterovirus, and bacterial gingivitis (see p. 135). All of these diseases are characterized by the simultaneous appearance of multiple aphthoid lesions. They do not show the typical protracted course with multiple recurrences of a few aphthae at a time.

Clinical Appearance

1. Recurrent aphthae are characterized by the sudden appearance of painful erosions approximately 3 to 4 mm in size that are covered by a white or yellowish fibrinous coating surrounded by an erythematous zone and that run a protracted course. In the beginning, the lesions often appear as nodules.
2. The disease involves mainly the mucous membranes of cheeks and lips, tongue, and gingivae.
3. Individual aphthae heal within a few days to 2 weeks. They recur in batches of a few aphthae at a time over a period of several months or even years.
4. Special forms include solitary aphthae, giant aphthae, simultaneous or alternately appearing genital aphthae, and very deep ulcerous aphthae (slowly healing over a period of several weeks or months). Consultation with an experienced dermatologist or stomatologist may be necessary to confirm the diagnosis and to exclude Behçet's and other diseases.
5. In some patients, Crohn's disease, ulcerative colitis, or a deficiency of iron, vitamin B_{12}, or folic acid is an underlying disorder.

Therapy

Treatment is still unsatisfactory. The therapeutic goal is reduction of pain and speedier healing of the lesions. Present-day treatment cannot prevent recurrences or prolong the symptom-free interval.

1. In most cases, the symptoms are minor and do not require treatment. The patients should not be burdened with a treatment that is more bothersome than the disease. Occasionally, a malt sucker can alleviate the symptoms.
2. Sour or spicy foods, citrus fruit, and alcoholic beverages can increase the discomfort and should be avoided. Mouthwash and toothpastes that cause pain should not be used.
3. Topical corticosteroid preparations can be beneficial in patients with extensive involvement and increased pain (sucking of Betnesol lozenges, 4 to 6 per day, where available). Application of adhesive creams with (Kenalog in Orabase) or without corticosteroids 3 times a day may also be helpful.
4. Topical application of anesthetic preparations may be indicated for severe pain (e.g., anesthetic lozenges). The accompanying temporary numbness of the surrounding area must be accepted. Topical antibiotic solutions or systemic antibiotics, cauterization with silver nitrate, and antiseptic solutions such as chlorhexidine or gentian violet solutions are not effective for treatment of recurrent aphthae.

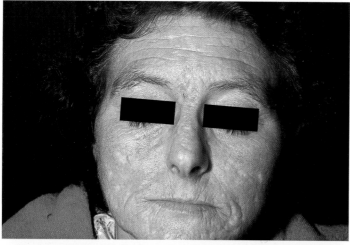

Figure 13. Artifact. White indented scars resulting from habitual excoriations in the face.

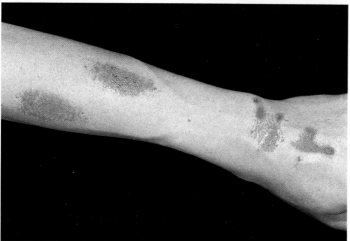

Figure 14. Artifact. Shallow fresh and old excoriations caused by repeated scraping with a kitchen knife.

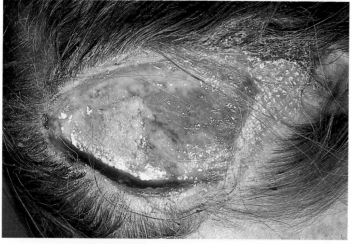

Figure 15. Artifact. Scalp defect caused by repeated trauma with a knife.

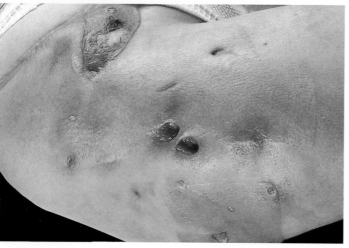

Figure 16. Artifact. Abscesses, fistulae, and their sequelae treated by multiple plastic surgical procedures in the right gluteal and thigh regions. Cause: Self injection of soapy solution into the subcutaneous tissue. The 18-year-old girl was hospitalized continuously in several hospitals for a period of 5 years before the cause could be found out.

Artifacts

Artifacts, self-inflicted skin lesions, are an aggressive expression of a psychologic disorder. The patients are frequently young or middle-aged women who are trying to attract attention or to derive benefits through these "artificial diseases." Often they are egocentric or love-starved persons. Only rarely do patients with self-inflicted lesions suffer from severe neurotic problems. Some patients, especially those with extensive self-inflicted wounds or self-mutilations, may be suffering from schizophrenia. Artifacts usually represent repeated injuries during a prolonged period of time. They are seldom solitary occurrences. The mechanisms of such artifacts are manifold. In most cases, they are due to mechanical trauma with knives or nails, or they are caused by acid or lye.

The diagnosis "artifact" should be made only in those cases in which self-infliction can be proved, which is often quite difficult. On direct inquiry, the patient rarely admits that the wound is self-inflicted. One must also keep in mind that the injuries can be inflicted unconsciously.

Clinical Appearance

1. The symptomatology depends on the mechanism of injury and can be manifold, such as contact dermatitis, circumscribed edemas, erosions, ulcers, and even deep abscesses. These lesions (e.g., erosions or ulcers) are often placed in a linear fashion or have sharp corners, in contrast to "natural diseases."
2. Artifacts are primarily located in areas the patient can reach with his or her own hands. We rarely find them on the back. They predominate on one side: in right-handed persons on the left, in left-handed persons on the right.

Therapy

1. Response to local treatment is usually prompt, provided further self-infliction can be prevented. Either the patient must be persuaded to stop these acts, or measures must be taken to prevent them, e.g., with starch bandages.
2. Psychiatric evaluation is necessary to exclude schizophrenia, endogenous or reactive depression, or neurotic disorders. In most patients, psychiatric evaluation will be negative, but conflict situations, which frequently exist, must be clarified and resolved. Several psychiatric sessions are usually necessary to discover and treat such conflict situations.

The prognosis for the treatment of artifacts is not very promising. The underlying problems are difficult to resolve, and recurrences are frequent. These patients have a tendency to change physicians to avoid discovery of their conflict situation.

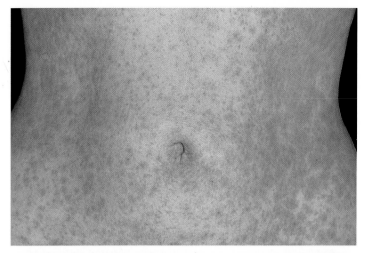

Figure 17. Maculopapular drug eruption of the trunk due to sulfamethoxydiazine.

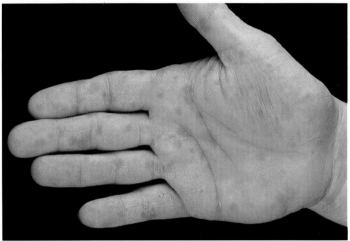

Figure 18. Macular drug eruption caused by Diclofenac. Typical appearance of the palm.

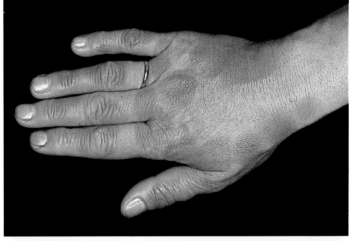

Figure 19. Macular drug eruption caused by Baralgin. Penny-size lesions on the dorsum of hand and fingers.

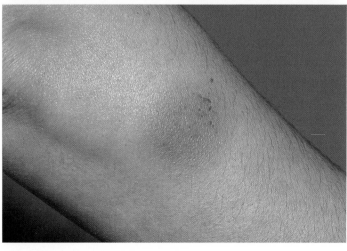

Figure 20. Fixed drug eruption. Brownish dusky discoloration with erythematous margin without central vesicular eruption. Caused by Metamizol.

Drug Eruptions

Undesired drug side effects frequently involve the skin. These symptoms are usually harmless and transient. Occasionally, however, they can develop into life-threatening systemic diseases, such as Lyell's disease (toxic epidermal necrolysis), anaphylactic symptoms with anaphylactic shock, or erythroderma. Symptomatology of drug side effects is extremely varied. The most frequent eruptions are spotty drug exanthemas, urticaria, drug-induced photosensitivity, drug-induced purpura, and itching. Less frequent reactions are fixed drug eruptions, skin discolorations, hair loss, nail disorders, and atrophy.

It is important to recognize these symptoms as adverse reactions to drugs and to determine which drugs are at fault. It must also be determined whether subsequent administration of the same or similar drugs will cause adverse reactions. The patient must be apprised of this, and the information must be entered on the patient's medical identification card.

Macular Exanthemas

Clinical Appearance

1. Macular or maculopapular exanthemas usually develop within the first 3 days following administration of the drug. Ampicillin exanthemas are exceptions. They normally develop 7 to 9 days after drug administration.
2. Clinically, drug eruptions can resemble infectious exanthemas, especially measles (morbilliform), German measles (rubelliform), or scarlet fever (scarlatiniform). The skin eruption alone is therefore not sufficient to warrant the diagnosis of drug reaction. The history and other symptoms must also be taken into consideration.
3. Fever (drug fever), enlarged lymph nodes, and eosinophilia are frequently concomitant symptoms of spotty exanthemas.
4. Progression into Lyell's disease (toxic epidermal necrolysis) (within hours) or into an erythroderma or exfoliative dermatitis (within days or weeks) is possible.

Differential Diagnosis

Macular drug eruptions must be differentiated from the spotty exanthemas of infectious diseases, food allergies, and intoxications.

Therapy

1. In most cases the symptoms are transient and not very pronounced. Systemic or local therapy is often not necessary.
2. Itching can be treated with systemic phenothiazine or another antihistamine (R.56, R.57), provided these drugs did not cause the eruption.
3. Other symptoms (fever, enlarged lymph nodes, arthralgia) may require systemic corticosteroid therapy (R.58).
4. The allergy must be entered on the patient's medical identification card to avoid future administration of this or similar drugs (cross-allergy).

Fixed Drug Eruptions

Clinical Appearance

1. One or more fairly large reddish-brown spots recur in the same location every time the drug is given. The formation of bullae is possible.
2. A typical residual brownish discoloration can persist at the site of the lesion for months or even years.

Therapy

The causative drug must be identified and eliminated from the patient's therapy. Bullae may be evacuated and dabbed with a disinfective iodine solution (R.17). No other treatment is necessary.

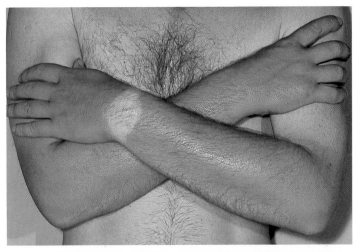

Figure 21. Phototoxic drug reaction, caused by Demeclocycline. Acute inflammatory erythema, limited strictly to the areas exposed to light.

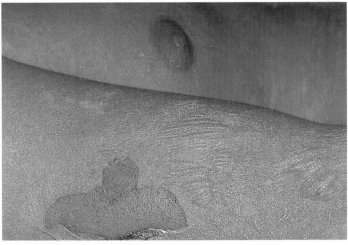

Figure 22. Lyell's syndrome. Extensive sloughing of the outer epidermal layers with erosions and bullae as in second degree burns.

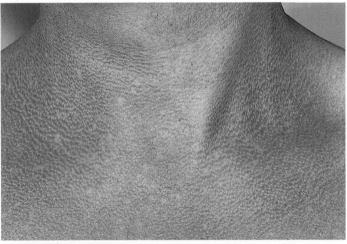

Figure 23. Cortisone skin with telangiectasias and brownish erythema between the follicles on the lower neck.

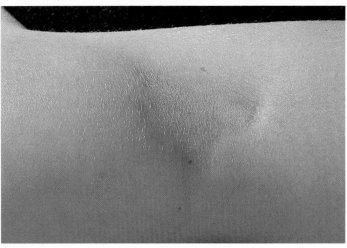

Figure 24. Lipoatrophy caused by inadvertent subcutaneous instead of intracutaneous injection of a corticosteroid crystal suspension.

Lyell's Syndrome (Toxic Epidermal Necrolysis)

Clinical Appearance

1. Influenza-like prodromal symptoms and a spotty skin eruption are followed by extensive sloughing of the epidermis, causing large erosions as in scalding.
2. General symptoms consist of pain and severe malaise, as well as symptoms resulting from the extensive loss of epidermis: circulatory failure with symptoms of shock, kidney failure, sepsis, and toxic damage to internal organs.
3. Late symptoms and sequelae are loss of hair and nails, pigmentation, and adhesions of the conjunctiva (symblepharon).

Therapy

The disease must be treated like a severe burn. The patient should be hospitalized for treatment, severe cases in the intensive care unit.

Light-Provoked Drug Reactions (see also pp. 89, 91)

Clinical Appearance

1. Erythema, scaling, occasional blistering, thickening of the skin, and itching are symptoms.
2. The eruptions are limited to skin areas exposed to light, such as the face and hands.

Therapy

1. The causative agent must be determined and its administration avoided.
2. Topical treatment with a corticosteroid-containing cream (for acute symptoms) or an ointment (for subacute and chronic changes) is appropriate.
3. Excessive exposure to light must be avoided until all symptoms have healed.
4. A sunscreen may be indicated.

Urticaria and Angioedema (see p. 141)

Urticaria is one of the most frequent drug eruptions of the skin. It can be either an allergic or a nonallergic reaction, and thus part of an anaphylactic or anaphylactoid reaction of the entire organism, and can then be associated with the symptomatology of shock. Urticaria is most frequently seen after administration of analgesics but can be caused by almost any medication. The causative agent must be avoided since the symptoms of allergic urticaria often increase in severity with repeated administration of the medication.

Clinical features and treatment will be discussed on p. 141.

Purpura (Hemorrhage into the Skin)

Hemorrhage into the skin can be caused by medication-induced allergic and nonallergic thrombocytopenia (cytostatic and analgesic drugs) and clotting disorders (cephalosporins).

Clinical Appearance

1. Depending on the severity of the disorder, one can see a variety of symptoms ranging from petechiae to extensive hemorrhage into the skin and mucous membranes.
2. Areas of skin exposed to mechanical forces are involved most often.

Therapy

Treatment is determined by the clotting and thrombocyte status and by the pathomechanics of the disorder. In severe cases, replacement of clotting factors or platelets, or both, may be necessary. Administration of corticosteroids may also be indicated.

Progressive pigment purpura ("Adalin purpura") and Schönlein's purpura are special forms with vascular involvement and a different clinical symptomatology.

Cortisone-Induced Skin Changes (Cortisone Skin)

Prolonged use of a corticosteroid-containing cream or ointment can produce local skin changes, such as erythema, thinning of the skin, increased hair growth, striae, and skin hemorrhage. Topical cortisone application over large areas of skin can lead to increased steroid absorption with generalized symptoms.

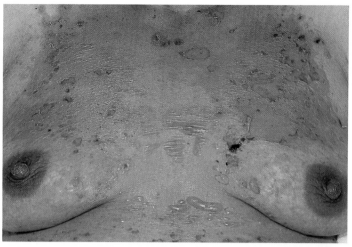

Figure 25. Pemphigus vulgaris. Flaccid bullae and extensive erosions on erythematous base.

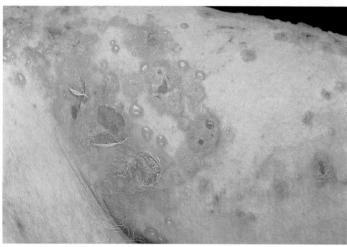

Figure 26. Pemphigus vulgaris, left thigh. Bullae originating on an initially normal skin, followed by erosions.

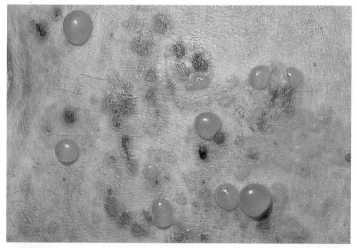

Figure 27. Bullous pemphigoid. Individual and crops of flaccid and tense bullae in various stages of development.

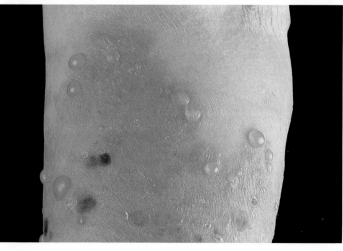

Figure 28. Bullous pemphigoid. Erythematous area with peripheral bullae and remnants of bullae on the flexor side of the left forearm.

Vesiculobullous Diseases

Bullae and vesicles are symptoms that can occur in diseases unrelated to one another, such as mosquito bites, contact dermatitis, erythema multiforme, and certain viral diseases (e.g., herpes simplex, herpes zoster).

The so-called vesiculobullous diseases are chronic diseases with generalized blistering. The patient may need to be hospitalized for a diagnostic workup that includes histologic and immunohistologic examinations, and in some instances electron microscope studies. The therapeutic program is usually determined during hospitalization.

Pemphigus Vulgaris

The disease is caused by the presence of autoantibodies to the intercellular junctions of the epidermis, making the junctions defective and leading to the formation of spontaneous or traumatic fissures and blisters.

Clinical Appearance

1. Blisters, remnants of blisters and erythema can be seen, occasionally with residual brown pigmentation.
2. The mucosa of the mouth is often involved; in more than 50 percent of the cases, this precedes the skin lesions.
3. There is a chronic course over many years with acute attacks of the disease. Without proper treatment the disease can be fatal.

Therapy

1. The disease responds promptly to systemic therapy with high doses of corticosteroids (R.58); this may be combined with immunosuppressors such as azathioprine or cyclophosphamide. After successful suppression of antibody formation, therapies are gradually reduced to a maintenance dose. Generally, therapy has to be continued for at least several months.
2. Topical treatment with antiseptics and corticosteroids is less important than is the systemic treatment.

Bullous Pemphigoid

This is the most frequently occurring of all blistering diseases and is seen most often in elderly individuals. The bullae are subepidermal and are caused by an antigen-antibody reaction along the basement membrane. The diagnosis is made by histologic and immunohistologic examinations of biopsy material.

Clinical Appearance

1. Bullous pemphigoid usually affects elderly patients and lasts many months or even years.
2. The disease is characterized by the appearance of bullae on normal skin or erythematous skin, which is raised as in urticaria. There is usually a mixture of tense bullae, remnants of bullae, erosions, erythema, and brownish discoloration. The patients frequently complain of unpleasant skin sensations ranging from itching to burning.
3. The oral mucosa is rarely involved.

Therapy

1. The disease usually responds well to high doses of corticosteroids that are later reduced to a maintenance dose. Corticosteroids may be supplemented with erythromycin or azathioprine.
2. Local therapy consists of evacuation of bullae and application of disinfectant solutions (R.17).

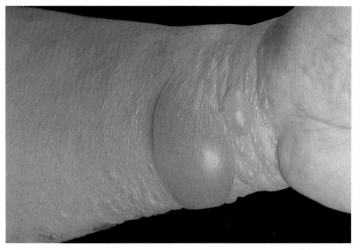

Figure 29. Bullous pemphigoid. Bullae and erosions of varying size on erythematous skin.

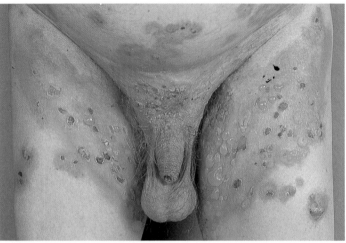

Figure 30. Dermatitis herpetiformis. Symmetric urticarial erythema with fresh and ruptured bullae. Circinate borders surround the lesions.

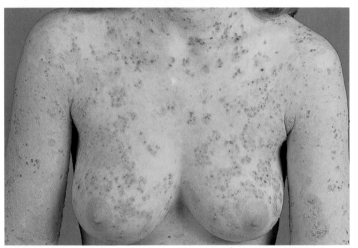

Figure 31. Dermatitis herpetiformis. Generalized, largely symmetric appearance of urticarial lesions. Formation of vesicles and crusts around the periphery of the lesions.

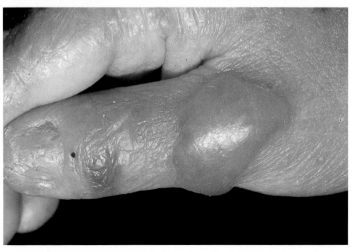

Figure 32. Epidermolysis bullosa hereditaria dystrophica. Formation of bullae in mechanically stressed or traumatized areas. Onychodystrophy is typical for this disease.

Dermatitis Herpetiformis

This is a chronic relapsing disease that lasts over many years or even decades. The cause is not clear. The diagnosis is confirmed histologically, and especially with characteristic immunohistologic findings that consist of IgA deposits in the upper corium.

Clinical Appearance

1. The clinical picture may be polymorphic. Frequently, symmetrically grouped or peripherally located vesicular lesions on urticarial erythema can be observed.
2. Subjectively, the patients complain of a burning sensation that is frequently more severe than itching.
3. Occasionally the oral mucosa is involved.
4. The patients are usually young or middle-aged. The disease rarely begins in old age.

Therapy

1. The treatment of choice for suppression of symptoms is prolonged systemic administration of dapsone in the lowest dose that will control the symptoms (usually 50 to 100 mg daily). Side effects of dapsone may be severe, so the patient and his or her laboratory tests must be monitored carefully.
2. Topical treatment consists of evacuation of blisters and application of antiseptic agents (R.17).
3. Strict adherence to a gluten-free diet may clear skin lesions or decrease dapsone requirements.

Epidermolysis Bullosa Hereditaria

This is a group of rare genetic disorders resulting from inadequate fixation of epidermis on the dermis. A mild blow, slight pressure, or shearing forces can lead to the formation of blisters. There are several subgroups that can be differentiated by clinical and electron microscope criteria. Mild forms of the disease occur more frequently.

Clinical Appearance

1. Formation of blisters and erosions occurs in areas in which the skin is exposed to mechanical forces. The soles of the feet, the hands, and areas of frequent contact with the environment are often involved.
2. The disease usually begins in early childhood and runs a prolonged course. Improvement of symptoms during adulthood is possible.

Therapy

Effective causative treatment of these genetically fixed diseases does not exist. Trauma should be avoided as much as possible, as well as increased heat (such as hot baths, which enhance the formation of blisters).

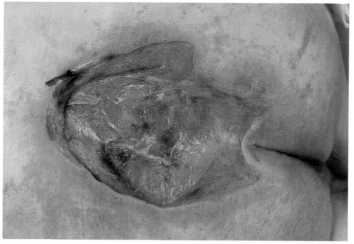

Figure 33. Deep sacral decubitus ulcer.

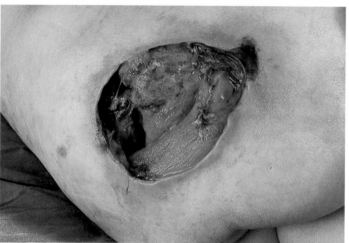

Figure 34. Decubitus ulcer, right hip. Deep ulcer with necrotic tissue and exposed musculature.

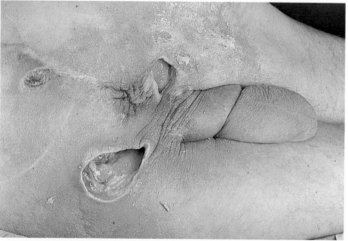

Figure 35. Decubitus ulcer in the gluteal region with extensive pocket formation. Ulcer and pockets were cleaned by appropriate nursing procedures.

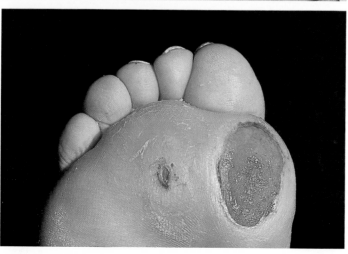

Figure 36. Malum perforans. Ulcers on the ball of the forefoot in a patient with polyneuropathy.

Decubitus

Decubitus ulcers occur as a result of pressure against individual areas of the body in patients who are unable to move adequately. This constant pressure produces atrophic changes and can lead to pressure necrosis. The patients are usually bedridden and suffering from generalized weakness and cachexia subsequent to chronic diseases, neurologic disorders, or severe disorders of the musculoskeletal system. Sensory changes can prevent normal physiologic shifts in position and result in decubitus ulcers. This occurs in diseases such as multiple sclerosis, paraplegia, and polyneuropathy (malum perforans of the ball of the great toe) and in comatose patients, e.g., those suffering from intoxication with barbiturates or other hypnotics. In these patients, a decubitus ulcer can develop within 1 or 2 days on the areas in contact with the bed. Patients with poorly developed subcutaneous fat are especially at risk.

Clinical Appearance

1. Erythema with occasional inflammatory infiltration can be seen. This skin becomes less resistant to shearing forces, and shearing can easily lead to detachment of the epidermis, with resultant erosions and shallow ulcers.
2. In hyperkeratotic areas, a decubital injury to the deeper layers of the skin initially causes a blister, which often becomes hemorrhagic.
3. Prolonged pressure may cause deep, purulent ulcers with undermined margins and fistulae followed by exposure of muscles, fasciae, tendons, and bone.
4. The ischemic changes are initially limited to the pressure areas, especially the sacral region, heels, and shoulders.

Therapy

General

The most important therapeutic measure is relief of pressure on the affected region. For sacral decubiti the patient must be maintained in a lateral or prone position. The use of decubitus mattresses, alternating air circulating mattresses, rotating frame beds, soft bedding, sheepskin, and so on, is important for even distribution of pressure. An additional prophylactic measure is the use of a blow dryer for periods of 10 minutes several times daily to areas of maceration. The skin regions at risk should be carefully massaged with ice cubes. Bland emollients are helpful when dry, fissured skin is present.

Systemic

It is important to improve the patient's general condition with tasty food, rich in calories, and good emotional care by the nursing staff.

External

Local therapy is secondary to relief of pressure and depends on the extent of the ulcer.

1. Erythema may require topical treatment with silicon spray or a soft zinc paste (R.28), in addition to pressure relief.
2. Erosions and shallow ulcers should be treated with normal wound care, such as disinfectant solutions (R.2, R.17), ointments (R.32), or dyes (R.14).
3. For deep ulcers and those with a thick coating, such measures for wound cleaning as wet dressings (R.1), debriding agents (R.41), and later medication to enhance the formation of granulation tissue are indicated. (See also p. 25.) Crusts and necrotic tissue should be removed mechanically as much as possible, followed by irrigation with H_2O_2 and disinfectant solutions. This may require the use of a bulbous cannula if the margin is undermined or if a fistula is present. Pockets or niches should be treated by irrigation and application of debriding agents.
4. Surgical procedures (excision of necrosis, coverage of defects by rotating flaps) can expedite healing of an ulcer but are usually indicated only in patients who will not be bedridden for the rest of their lives.

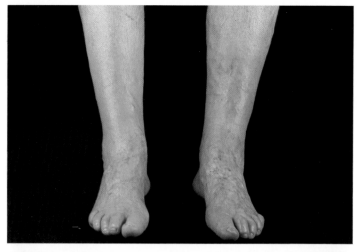

Figure 37. Arterial occlusive disease. Condition following arterial embolus of the left leg several days ago. Bluish discoloration of the toes.

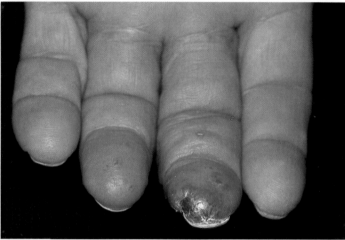

Figure 38. Arterial occlusive disease. Necrosis of the tip of the third finger, beginning necrosis of the tip of the fourth finger, left hand.

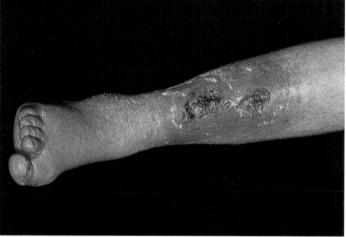

Figure 39. Leg ulcer in a patient with arterial occlusive disease. Typical location in the middle of the lower leg.

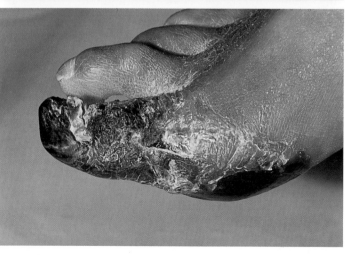

Figure 40. Diabetic gangrene. Dry gangrene of the big toe. The toe is almost mummified.

Vascular Disorders

Arterial Occlusive Diseases

The causes of arterial occlusion are manifold. The blood supply can be cut off by tight bandages. It can be obstructed by arterial occlusive disease, which can be a complication of diabetes mellitus; by deposits on the vessel walls, with resulting narrowing of the lumen; or by acute occlusion caused by arterial thrombi or drugs such as adrenaline, noradrenaline, or ergotamine preparations. Acute arterial occlusions require immediate hospitalization and treatment. The practicing physician encounters arterial occlusive disease more frequently as a chronic vascular disorder with reduction of blood supply to the heart (coronary heart disease), kidneys, brain, abdominal organs, and legs.

Clinical Appearance

Peripheral arterial occlusive disease can be subdivided into four clinical stages.

> *Stage 1:* No symptoms. The occlusion can be diagnosed only by angiography or occasionally by Doppler examination.
>
> *Stage 2:* Pain on exercise. Increased oxygen demand by the musculature produces pain with intermittent claudication. The pain free walking distance depends on the degree of vascular obstruction.
>
> *Stage 3:* Resting pain. Blood supply is impaired to the degree that pain is present even at rest. For relief of pain, the patient often lets his or her leg hang out of the bed.
>
> *Stage 4:* In addition to the previous symptoms, necroses develop in the areas with impaired blood supply.

The skin is usually involved only in arterial occlusive disorders of Stage 4 or in acute complete arterial obstruction.

Thin, dry, pale skin of the legs, as well as reduced skin temperature and hair loss, is often an indication that blood supply to that region is impaired.

Therapy

It is extremely important to eliminate all risk factors as early as possible (lack of exercise, smoking, arterial hypertension, diabetes mellitus, disorders of fat metabolism, and gout). Vascular training with exercise therapy is useful in Stages 1 and 2. Combined arterial and venous disorders, which are frequently present in older patients, are more difficult to treat. Compression would impair arterial blood supply even more. In Stages 2, 3, and 4, it must also be determined whether a circumscribed stenosis can be removed surgically or by catheter dilatation. In more advanced stages, amputation of the involved extremity is often the last resort. Surgery is indicated when moist gangrene with impending sepsis is present or when pain is so severe that it can no longer be relieved with medication.

Systemic

Drug therapy with vasodilating substances (caution: "steal phenomenon," that is, reduction of blood supply in the involved region through redistribution of blood), rheologic drugs, drugs that prevent thrombocyte aggregation, or anticoagulants is less important in comparison with the previously mentioned therapeutic measures.

External

Topical therapy should prevent infection of necroses. Dressings can produce moist chambers with anaerobic infection and should be avoided. Treatment with dry powders and disinfectant solutions is preferable until the necroses are demarcated. Mechanical removal of necroses must be done with great care to avoid additional tissue damage.

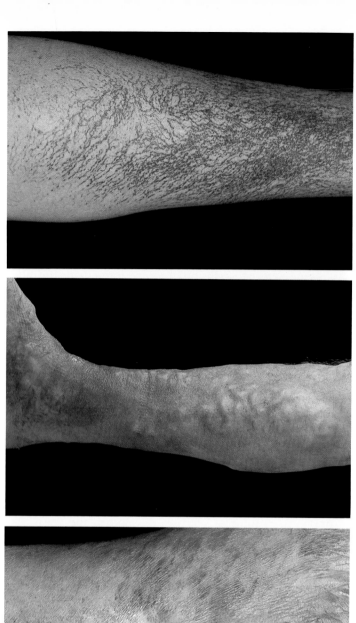

Figure 41. Fans of intracutaneous varices of the lower leg.

Figure 42. Varicose veins caused by insufficiency of the greater saphenous vein.

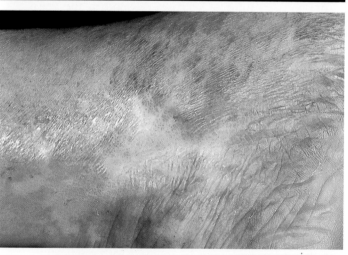

Figure 43. Capillaritis alba in chronic venous insufficiency. Circumscribed white sclerotic foci with punctate blood vessels, left medial malleolar area.

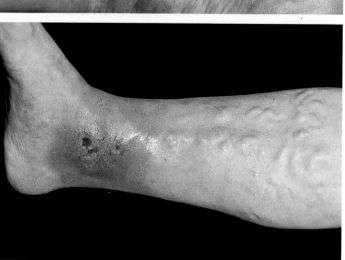

Figure 44. Venous leg ulcer in a patient with chronic venous insufficiency. Several ulcers in the area of the medial malleolus. Dermatosclerosis, deposition of hemosiderin. Massive varicosis.

Venous Disorders; Ulcus Cruris (Leg Ulcer)

Statistical studies have shown that approximately 20 percent of all citizens of the Federal Republic of Germany have varicoses of the saphenous system. Approximately 1 million patients are suffering from venous leg ulcers, and there are some 16,000 fatal pulmonary emboli annually, most of which are due to thromboses of the leg veins. These figures show the significant impact of disorders of the leg veins. In addition to a familial disposition, there are individual factors such as being overweight, a predominantly sitting or standing occupation, the wrong footwear (elimination of the calf muscle pump by high heels) and hormonal factors such as ovulation inhibitors and pregnancy that can be responsible for manifestation of the disorder. Women are afflicted more frequently than are men; incidence and severity of symptoms are higher in the older age groups. The causes of chronic leg vein insufficiency include primary varicoses, recurrent thrombophlebitis, primary insufficiency of the perforating veins, and prior thrombophlebitis. Dermatologic symptoms develop independently of the causes of chronic leg vein insufficiency.

Clinical Appearance

1. One of the earliest symptoms is the patient's complaint of "heavy legs." The earliest dermatologic sign of chronic incompetence is edema of the ankles, which initially occurs in the evening after prolonged standing and in hot weather.
2. Varices occur at the same time or somewhat later. These can be fan-shaped, intracutaneous varices (purely cosmetic), reticular varices, or varices of the saphenous system (v. saphena magna or v. saphena parva), depending on the size of the involved veins.
3. Persisting edemas lead to protein deposition in the interstitium, with increased formation of connective tissue. The skin is firm and difficult to impress (dermatosclerosis).
4. Prolonged stasis can lead to extravasation of erythrocytes (stasis purpura). Hemoglobin is metabolized into hemosiderin, which remains in the tissues for a long time and causes brown discoloration of the skin.
5. Incompetence of the perforating veins often produces capillaritis alba distal to their point of entry. These are whitish areas of atrophic scarring that develop without trauma, usually in the ankle region.
6. Increasing nutritional disturbance of the skin frequently leads to leg ulcers, either spontaneously or as a result of minimal trauma, erysipelas, or thrombophlebitis.
7. Areas of predilection for venous leg ulcers are the ankle region and the distal part of the lower leg.
8. The morphology of venous leg ulcers is manifold. It includes small, shallow ulcers that are often painful and that develop on the basis of capillaritis alba, as well as ulcers involving the lower leg in a sleeve-like fashion and developing as a result of extensive thrombotic obstruction of varicose skin veins.
9. The development of a squamous cell carcinoma is a rare complication, occurring in long-standing ulcers (after decades). Rapidly proliferating granulation tissue is a suspicious finding and should be examined histologically.

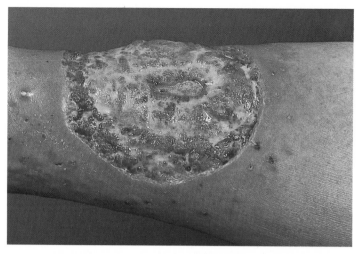

Figure 45. Venous leg ulcer in a patient with post-thrombotic syndrome.

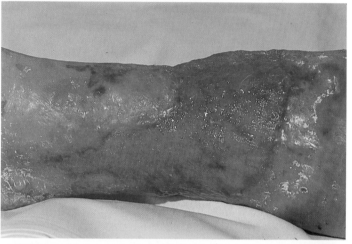

Figure 46. Venous leg ulcer. Severe post-thrombotic syndrome with extensive cufflike ulcer.

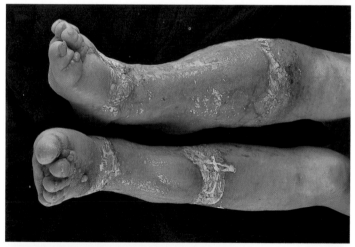

Figure 47. Cufflike ulcers on both lower legs in a patient with chronic venous insufficiency. Characteristic persistent edema of the forefoot and extensive, partially hyperkeratotic papillomatosis.

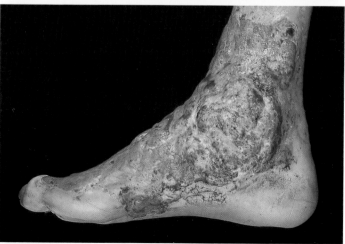

Figure 48. Squamous cell carcinoma on a venous leg ulcer that had persisted for 12 years (in a patient with generalized morphea).

Therapy

General

Exact phlebologic diagnosis is necessary before optimal long-term therapy can be established. Of primary importance is correction of the impaired venous blood flow. There are three ways to achieve this: compression therapy (see p. 241), injection with sclerosing solutions, and vein stripping. These methods complement each other to a certain degree, or they overlap for certain indications. In addition, specific dermatologic therapy may be necessary for the accompanying cutaneous symptoms, especially leg ulcers. The previously mentioned therapeutic measures may have to be supplemented by systemic drug treatment. Since chronic stasis conditions have a tendency to develop sensitization reactions, the routine use of most OTC ointments should be avoided. Contact allergies to the medications, preservatives, or bases contained in these ointments often develop and may make topical treatment of an ulcer very difficult at a later date. Exercises such as swimming, bicycling, or running are useful to enhance the musculovenous pump. Proper footwear with low heels is also important.

External

Topical therapy of leg ulcers is carried out in several stages: cleansing, promotion of granulation tissue, and epithelial coverage.

1. Disinfecting leg bath, e.g., with the addition of potassium permanganate, and the application of moist compresses with physiologic saline solution or aseptic solutions (R.2) is helpful.
2. Necrotic tissue should be removed with debriding medications (R.41). These medications can be applied in combination with moist compresses or the necrotic tissue can be removed with a curette (which may be painful).
3. Heavy fibrinous or necrotic coatings always contain bacteria. They should be removed to eliminate the growth medium for bacteria. Significant bacterial infection requiring local or systemic antibiotic treatment occurs rarely with venous leg ulcers.
4. Porous foam rubber materials have been developed for occlusive or semiocclusive dressings that may debride, promote granulation tissue, or speed epithelial migration, or a combination of these, especially when they are applied with mild pressure.

   Examples are Op-Site Bioclusive, Vigilon, and Duoderm. Contrary to mixed ointments, which often contain neomycin or balsam of Peru, these materials very rarely cause contact allergies. These dressings can be left in place for several days to avoid damage to the newly formed epithelial tissue by daily dressing changes.
5. Once clean granulations are present, antimicrobial powder (R.12) will promote granulation and epithelialization.
6. Application of a compression bandage (see p. 241) and mobilization of the patient are absolutely necessary as part of the therapeutic program. Compression bandages achieve their optimal effect only when the patient is ambulatory.
7. Large ulcers should be debrided and covered with split skin grafts according to Reverdin's or Meshgraft technique to shorten the healing time.
8. The patient should be referred to a phlebologist who is equipped to perform a thorough diagnostic workup before a decision is made whether prolonged compression therapy, injection with a sclerosing solution, or vein stripping is indicated.

Systemic

Systemic medications cannot replace the previously mentioned therapeutic measures for chronic leg vein insufficiency; they can only supplement them in individual cases. Diuretics can be useful to treat edema but are not recommended for the prophylaxis of edema. Medications to increase the venous tone may be helpful. These include dihydroergotamine, which, however, may damage the arterial blood flow (ergotism), and rheologic drugs (pentoxifylline, Dusodril, or Bufedil), as well as drugs that "seal" blood vessels, such as horse chestnut extract or Benzaron (where available).

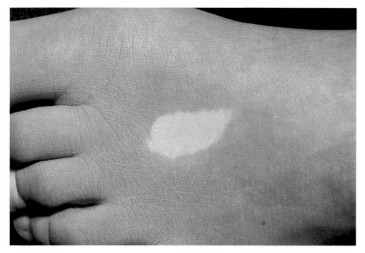

Figure 49. Acrocyanosis. Iris phenomenon (that is, blanching on finger pressure with subsequent retrograde blood flow), beginning in the periphery like an iris closing its diaphragm.

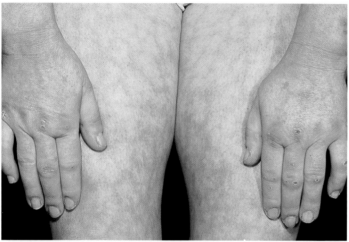

Figure 50. Livedo reticularis. Reticulate dusky vascular markings.

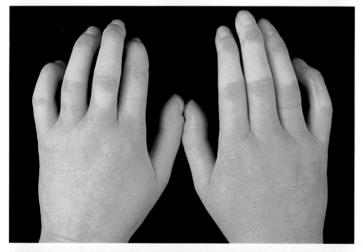

Figure 51. Raynaud's phenomenon. Blanching of the fingers induced by cold.

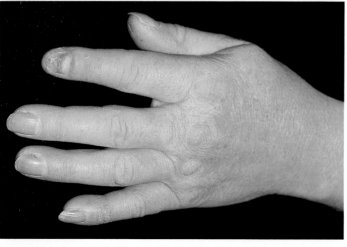

Figure 52. Raynaud's phenomenon. Phase of venous atonia with edematous swelling and mild cyanosis. Candidal infection of nail and nailbed, secondary to the impaired blood supply.

Other Common Vascular Disorders

These are primarily diseases of the small vessels that have an abnormal reaction to cold in common. The clinical severity of these disorders varies from functional problems (acrocyanosis) to severe illnesses, such as Raynaud's disease.

Acrocyanosis

Clinical Appearance

1. Poorly defined bluish-red discolorations of the acra, frequently associated with hyper-hidrosis. The so-called "iris-phenomenon" is of diagnostic importance.
2. The symptoms are found in the hands and feet and occasionally in the arms, legs, nose, and cheeks. In obese patients, gluteal area and mammae may be involved. Sometimes, there are transitions to chilblains (see p. 61).
3. The cold, moist hands and feet are often conspicuous; occasionally, there are complaints of paresthesias. These patients have a disposition for other skin diseases, such as warts (see p. 199), fungus infections (see pp. 105–111), and pyodermas (see p. 123–127). Acrocyanosis occurs mainly during puberty and almost always in women. The disorder disappears spontaneously after a few years and is no longer present in middle-aged persons.

Therapy

Vascular training with contrast baths, sauna, and athletic activities is important. Nicotine must be avoided.

Systemic

Drugs to improve blood supply and increase the tone of the vessel walls are often prescribed. Their effect in acrocyanosis, however, is questionable.

External

Protection from cold is very important.

Livedo Reticularis

Clinical Appearance

There is reticulated bluish discoloration of the skin on the arms, legs, and trunk that increases with exposure to cold (cutis marmorata). These symptoms develop in infants and adolescents, especially in females. It is questionable whether this represents a genuine disease process.

Raynaud's Disease, Raynaud's Phenomenon

The disorder is characterized by intermittent spasms of the small arteries of the fingers and toes, mainly as a result of exposure to cold. It occurs especially in the winter months. A number of causes have been identified, including diseases such as progressive sclero-derma, lupus erythematosus, cold agglutinin disease, cryoglobulinemia, vibration injuries, chemicals (PVC), or drugs (ergotamine, bleomycin).

Conditions whose cause cannot be identified are classified as Raynaud's disease. The disease occurs more frequently in women than in men. Prognosis is determined primarily by the underlying causative mechanism.

Clinical Appearance

Sudden blanching of several or all fingers will occur on exposure to cold. After a few minutes, a dark cyanotic discoloration occurs and gradually changes to a long-lasting red color (reactive hyperemia). These attacks can occur several times a day, depending on the severity of the disease.

Therapy

It is important to treat the underlying cause. Measures must be taken to protect against cold (mittens, muff, pocket heater). Smoking is prohibited.

Systemic

Calcium channel blockers (e.g., nifedipine 10 to 20 mg daily) can be used. Other "blood vessel active" drugs are less effective.

Topical

Nitrates (e.g., Nitrol ointment) have proven effective but should be used with caution.

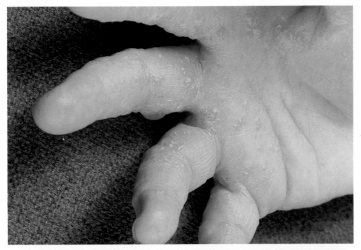

Figure 53. Dyshidrosis of the hand. Vesicle formation mainly on the sides of the fingers and in the palm of the hand.

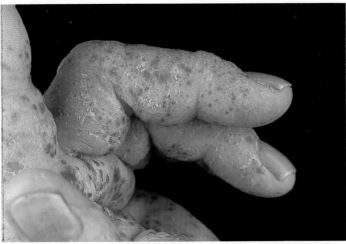

Figure 54. Dyshidrosis of the hand. Acute crop of vesicles with hemorrhage into the vesicles.

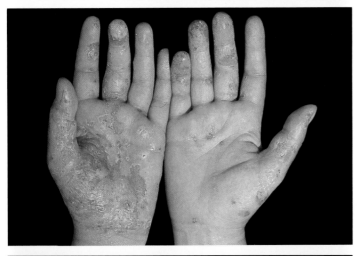

Figure 55. Dyshidrosis of the hand. Many intact and broken vesicles as well as erosions on the palms of both hands.

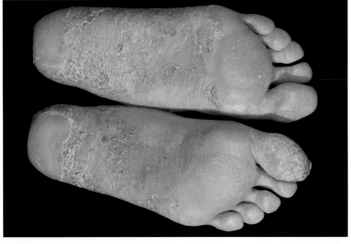

Figure 56. Dyshidrosis of the foot. Formation of vesicles, erythema, and scaling mainly on the sole of the foot.

Dyshidrosis

Pompholyx

This disease is characterized by recurrent vesicular eruptions on the sides of the fingers and toes as well as on their palmar and plantar surfaces. The cause remains obscure in most cases. Hot weather and high humidity favor dyshidrosis. In some patients, dyshidrosis is a symptom of atopic eczema; occasionally, it is due to a contact allergy or chronic nonallergic contact eczema (see p. 33) Dyshidrosis can occur acutely, with exacerbation of a stasis eczema of the lower legs, or very rarely as an accompanying symptom of dermatophytosis. Mechanical stress and work in a moist environment can increase the symptoms. In adults, dyshidrosis can occasionally develop into chronic hyperkeratotic eczema of the palms of the hands and the soles of the feet (see p. 43). Abortive forms occur frequently. The disease can also occur in children. It is sometimes difficult to differentiate it from psoriasis or palmoplantar pustulosis.

Clinical Appearance

1. The disorder is characterized by the sudden appearance of severely itching nodules that rapidly change into vesicular lesions. The vesicles can heal with desquamation. Occasionally, bullae form that can be very firm and painful, especially under the thick horny layer of the palm of the hand and the sole of the foot. These lesions often develop into weeping, painful erosions.
2. The lesions are characteristically located on the sides of the fingers and toes, especially at the transition line between the keratotic skin of the palmar or plantar side and the thinner dorsal skin. The palm of the hand and the sole of the foot can also be affected. Involvement is usually symmetric. Not infrequently, only the hands are affected.
3. Lymphangitis with painful swelling of the regional lymph nodes often complicates the disorder.
4. Hyperhidrosis is often a concomitant symptom.
5. Sometimes, only one attack occurs, but there can also be frequent relapses. The condition may persist for several months or many years.

Therapy

At the present time, there is no satisfactory treatment, especially for the chronic form.

1. Moist dressings (R.1) with disinfectant solutions (R.2) and corticosteroid creams (R.36b) are indicated when erosions predominate. Bullae are punctured to relieve pressure and pain. The skin of the bullae is left in place for protection against infection. Fatty ointments must be avoided.

   In subacute and chronic conditions, painting with a tar containing solution may be helpful (R.16).
2. Hand baths, e.g., with oak bark extract (tannic acid), are sometimes useful.
3. Systemic administration of antihistamines (R.56, R.57) may reduce itching. Systemic corticosteroids can suppress an acute attack, but the disease usually recurs after the medication is discontinued. Corticosteroids should be reserved for very severe conditions.
4. In a persistent disease with a chronic course, photochemotherapy (PUVA) can be successful. The patient should be referred to a dermatologist who has experience with this treatment modality.
5. Rubber or vinyl gloves should be used for work with water (dishes, cleaning) or with strong irritants (floor or household cleaners). These gloves should be worn over thin cotton gloves and not directly on the skin.

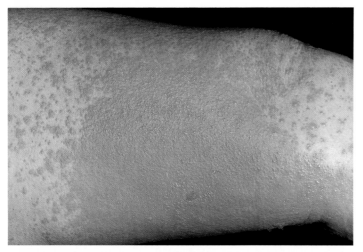

Figure 57. Acute allergic contact dermatitis caused by an ointment for chilblains. Erythema, papules, vesicles, and central erosion with ill-defined borders on the right thigh.

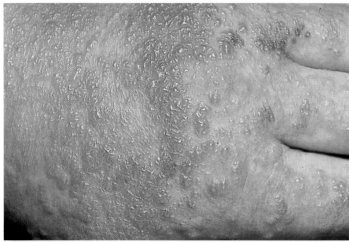

Figure 58. Acute contact dermatitis caused by benzoyl peroxide. Vesicular stage.

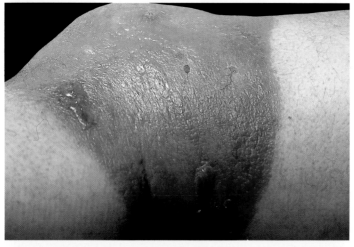

Figure 59. Acute allergic contact dermatitis caused by heparin ointment. Erythema and vesicles, some of which are hemorrhagic. The lesion is sharply delineated.

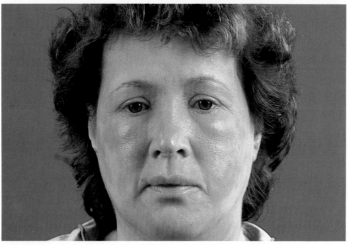

Figure 60. Acute contact dermatitis, caused by shampoo. Erythema and marked edema.

Eczematous Diseases

Individual eczematous diseases can be differentiated from one another by their clinical symptoms and the course of the disease. A contact eczema is usually due to contact with an injurious substance. Nonallergic contact eczemas occur much more frequently than do allergic ones, especially chronic nonallergic contact eczema, which results from repeated exposure to toxic substances over a long period of time. Acute contact eczema is due to substances that primarily irritate the skin, such as alkali or wound secretions. Some eczemas, like diaper rash and stasis eczema on the lower legs of patients with venous insufficiency, may be considerably influenced by external factors. Other eczematous diseases are caused primarily or exclusively by endogenous factors such as seborrheic eczema, pityriasis alba, juvenile papular dermatitis, nummular eczema, chronic hyperkeratotic eczema of hands or feet, ear eczema, lichen simplex chronicus, and atopic dermatitis.

Acute Allergic Contact Eczema

The patient must be sensitized by previous exposure to contact allergens, such as plants (poison ivy, primrose, chrysanthemum), textiles (dyes, rubber substitutes), topical medications (antibiotics, balsam of Peru), and many industrial materials (chromium salts, resins). The capacity of the individual substances to sensitize varies. Children under the age of 10 years rarely develop allergic contact eczema. They do, however, develop nonallergic eczema. The same is true for older patients.

Clinical Appearance

1. Erythema, nodules, vesicles, bullae, erosions, weeping surfaces, and crusts characterize an acute contact eczema. All these symptoms can occur simultaneously. At other times, one or more symptoms may be present. The patient usually complains of marked itching. With pronounced facial involvement, edema of the lids and periorbital region also develops.
2. Symptoms evolve slowly, at least several hours but usually 1 to 3 days following contact with the causative agent. The lesions heal within 2 to 3 weeks.
3. Frequently, the affected area corresponds to the area in contact with the allergen, but occasionally it exceeds the contact area.
4. Disseminated reactions are possible with rapidly developing scattered nodules that exceed the contact area and also involve other regions of the body.

Therapy

It is important to identify and eliminate the causative agent, especially by history and patch test.

1. Moist dressings (R.1) are the treatment of choice for acute weeping contact eczema or contact dermatitis. In addition, corticosteroid–containing creams (R.36b, c) can be applied thinly.
2. For nonweeping lesions, a shake mixture (R.20) or topical corticosteroids (creams) (R.36) can be used for short periods (no longer than 2 weeks).
3. Antihistamines are useful for relief of pruritus (R.56, R.57). A brief treatment period with systemic corticosteroids does not shorten the healing period but may be justified in severe cases (R.58).

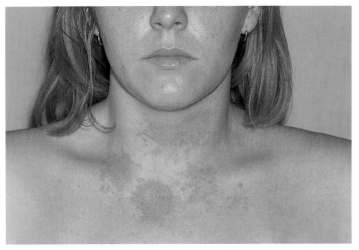

Figure 61. Allergic contact dermatitis caused by custom jewelry in a patient sensitized to nickel.

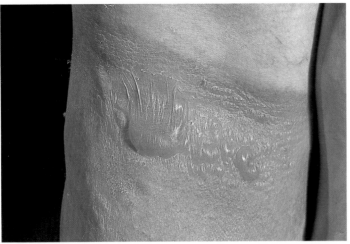

Figure 62. Acute allergic contact dermatitis caused by stocking dye. Erythema and blisters in the left popliteal area.

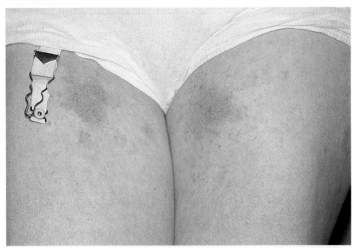

Figure 63. Allergic nickel dermatitis caused by the patient's garters. Ill-defined papular dermatitis.

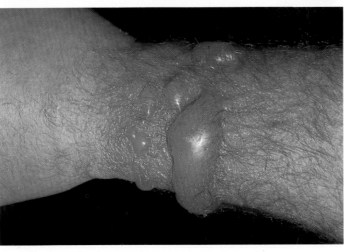

Figure 64. Bullous allergic contact dermatitis caused by ichthyol-containing ointment: right forearm.

Chronic Allergic Contact Eczema

This is an eczema caused and maintained by prolonged exposure to contact allergens, such as nickel (jewelry), rubber (underwear, gloves), or leather (shoes).

Clinical Appearance

1. Pruritus, thickening of the skin, coarse surface markings, occasionally hyperkeratosis, and rhagades are the symptoms of chronic allergic contact eczema. There is frequent recurrence of acute eczematization, with papules and crust formation.
2. Healing occurs slowly and with scaling. Sometimes, permanent pigmentation remains.

Therapy

Recognition and elimination of the contact allergen are important for a successful treatment.

1. Corticosteroid-containing creams and ointments (R.36) shorten the course of the disease significantly.
2. Tar or urea-containing ointments in combination with corticosteroids (R.37b, d, e) are useful for thickened and lichenified lesions.
3. Protective ointments (R.31b, c) are indicated for prophylaxis of occupational contact allergies.

Chronic, Nonallergic Contact Eczema (Cumulative Toxic Contact Dermatitis)

This is an important and common form of eczema. Constant contact with weak caustic solutions, concentrated detergents, organic solvents or occasionally just plain water can cause damage of the skin. The skin reacts to this chronic toxic irritation with chronic eczema. This is observed frequently in housewives, members of medical and paramedical professions, cleaning and kitchen personnel (damage from water and detergents), brick layers (damage from alkali), and other building occupations. It occurs frequently in patients with atopic dermatitis. A contact allergy can develop secondarily.

Clinical Appearance

The symptoms resemble those of chronic eczema.

1. Dryness and thinning of the skin with fissures, scaling, rhagades, and itching are seen. Later, the skin thickens, and skin markings become coarse. There is recurrent acute eczematization with dyshidrotic vesicles, erosions, and crusts (see p. 31).
2. The symptoms are limited to the region exposed to the chronic trauma, almost exclusively the hands. Normally, disseminated reactions do not occur.
3. Irritability of the skin is increased. Even minor trauma or psychic stress can increase the eczema.

Therapy

1. The most important measures are recognition and elimination of the causes. Housewives should avoid working with water or with strong irritants (floor and household cleaners) and should wear vinyl gloves over cotton gloves.
2. Topical therapy consists of the application of ointments containing corticosteroids (R.36), urea (R.37b), or tar substances (R.37e). (No occlusive dressings.)
3. Skin-protective ointments can be used prophylactically.
4. It is important that the patient gets enough sleep.
5. Systemic treatment with corticosteroids or antihistamines is usually not necessary.

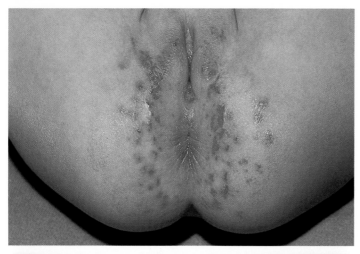

Figure 65. Diaper rash. Erosive nodules in the perianal area.

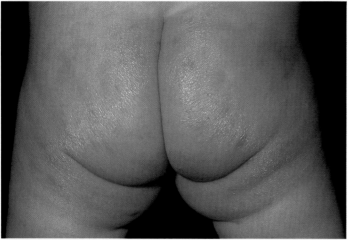

Figure 66. Diaper rash. Erythema, mild scaling, and papules. Symmetric distribution in the gluteal area.

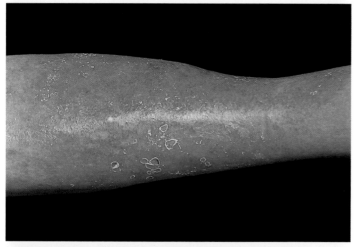

Figure 67. Stasis dermatitis in a patient with chronic venous insufficiency. Erythema and scaling, right lower leg.

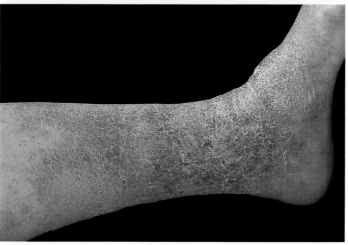

Figure 68. Stasis dermatitis in a patient with chronic venous insufficiency. Considerable scaling, brownish discoloration, and erosions on the lower leg and dorsum of the foot—most pronounced in the malleolar area.

Eczema due to Secondary Contact Sensitization

A long-term nonallergic eczema is present initially (eczema of the lower legs in patients with chronic venous insufficiency, chronic nonallergic contact eczema, long-standing dyshidrosis, or chronic hyperkeratotic eczema of the palms and soles of the feet). This causes increased permeability of the skin and secondary contact allergy. In addition to the primary eczema, sensitization to the contact material (topical medications or metal ions such as chromates or nickel) occurs. With renewed contact, these allergens can cause allergic contact eczema. Sensitization can be demonstrated with patch tests. Contact sensitization with positive patch test reactions, however, is in many of these cases only a secondary manifestation and is not responsible for the chronic nature of the eczema.

Diaper Dermatitis, Diaper Eczema

Diaper dermatitis develops in the region in contact with the diaper as a result of skin irritation from decomposition products of urine and feces, especially in infants with diarrhea or as a result of poor care and in children whose diapers are not changed often enough. Candida infection is superimposed on long-standing diaper eczema almost regularly.

Clinical Appearance

1. Erythema, nodules, and occasionally weeping surfaces are characteristic clinical findings.
2. The symptoms originate in the anal and genital regions. Initially they are limited to areas in contact with the diaper. With severe involvement and in cases secondarily infected with Candida, the lesions can spread to other areas of the skin (satellite lesions).
3. In long-standing cases, nodules and prurigo-like nodes often predominate. General well-being is usually impaired very little.

Therapy

1. The involved region must be kept dry; frequent diaper changes are important. Diapers should be left off for several hours during the day. Absorbent diapers must be used. Plastic pants should be avoided.
2. There should be careful removal of all urine and stool rests with oil and frequent baths. After the bath, the baby must be dried well and powdered.
3. Zinc oxide pastes (R.27) are effective.
4. Diarrhea must be treated. Fruit acids, especially fresh sour fruit must be avoided until the dermatitis is healed. Bananas can be given instead. Intestinal *Candida* infection must be treated (reservoir of organisms) (see p. 109).

Stasis Eczema, Stasis Dermatitis

Acute or chronic eczema of the lower leg can be found in patients with chronic venous insufficiency. Other symptoms, such as varices, pigmentation, dermatosclerosis, and so on, are also usually present (see p. 23).

Clinical Appearance

1. Erythema, nodules, scaling, sometimes with weeping and crust formation, are characteristic of stasis eczema.
2. Large bullae can be found in areas, with excessive and rapidly developing edema ("tension blisters," also in patients with cardiac edema).
3. Characteristic locations are the distal parts of the lower legs, the ankle region, and occasionally the dorsum of the foot. In prolonged conditions, the entire lower legs can be involved.
4. Bilateral involvement is seen frequently.

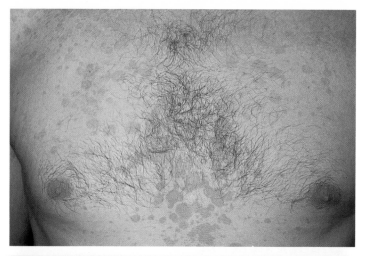

Figure 69. Seborrheic dermatitis. Yellowish-brown, sharply delineated, round lesions with scaling in the middle of the chest.

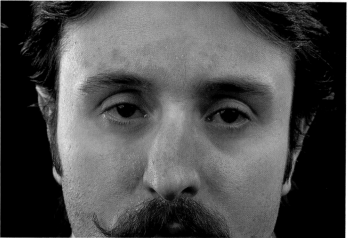

Figure 70. Seborrheic dermatitis. Erythema and scaling in the moustache and nasolabial area, eyebrows, and forehead.

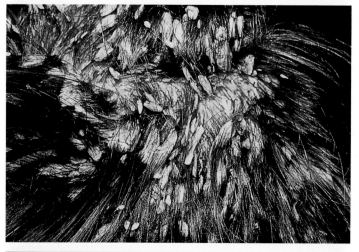

Figure 71. This sheathlike coating of the hairs can occur in patients with squamous diseases of the scalp such as seborrheic dermatitis and psoriasis. So-called "tinea amiantacea."

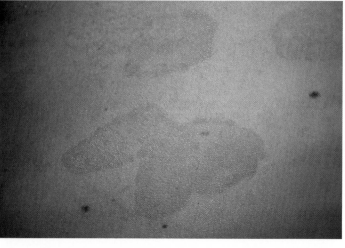

Figure 72. Seborrheic dermatitis. Flat, yellowish-brown, sharply delineated lesions on the trunk with mild scaling.

Therapy

1. The most important goal is elimination of the underlying edema by compression with elastic bandages, elastic stockings (see p. 241), and intermittent elevation of the involved extremity. This can be supplemented initially with a mild diuretic and with other phlebologic measures (see p. 25).
2. Topical therapy consists of moist dressings (3 times daily for 20 minutes) and corticosteroid-containing creams or pastes (R.30b, R.36b) to ease itching and reduce the other symptoms.
3. Other additives except corticosteroids should not be used for topical therapy to avoid secondary contact sensitization to these substances (such as local antibiotics). Local disinfectants and antibiotics are not necessary for treatment of stasis eczema.

Seborrheic Eczema

Seborrheic eczema can be found in several typical locations and subvarieties. It occurs mainly in areas with increased activity of sebaceous glands, especially the scalp, face, and chest, and less frequently in the axillae and the pubic region. In children, seborrheic eczema occurs only until the fourth month of life, probably on the basis of maternal hormones. Adults with light skin are afflicted more often. It has to be kept in mind that seborrheic eczema on the face occurs frequently in patients with AIDS.

Clinical Appearance

1. *Scalp.* Increased desquamation (a few noninflammatory scales are normal!), itching, and occasionally moderate erythema in individual patches or affecting the entire scalp. (The forehead can sometimes be involved for a distance of 1 cm, creating a band of eczema below the margin of the hair.) There can be significant itching. Scratching can produce erosions and crusts. Physical exertion and emotional stress increase the symptoms.
2. *Face.* Bandlike or patchy involvement in and between the eyebrows and nasolabial folds, and in the vicinity of the eyelashes. In men, the bearded area can also be involved. In other parts of the face, in and behind the ear, one occasionally finds erythema and desquamation, frequently with minimal itching.
3. *Chest.* The central area of the chest can be involved, with a few light brown or yellowish-red, sharply delineated, slightly scaling patches without a raised margin. Itching is usually absent. The lesions do not cause any subjective discomfort.

Therapy

1. The scalp should be washed with antiseborrheic shampoo two to three times per week. The shampoos should contain pyrithion-zinc (R.10b) or tar substances (R.10a) and should be allowed to take effect for several minutes. For erythematous changes, corticosteroid-containing tinctures can be useful (R.18). They must be applied to the scalp (1 drop every 3 to 4 cm). The hair is parted every 2 cm, and the tincture applied until the entire skin of the scalp has been treated. If these measures are unsuccessful, application of Keralyt scalp ointment may be indicated. The ointment should be rinsed out with a shampoo the next morning.
2. Lesions of the face and chest should be treated with corticosteroid-containing topicals, especially creams (R.36a) for several days until they are healed. Patients with seborrheic eczema rarely tolerate ointments or fatty externa except on the scalp.
   Caution: No long-term topical corticosteroid therapy of the face! It can cause erythema, atrophy, and rosacea-like symptoms. (See p. 131.)
3. Systemic therapy is not necessary. Effective therapeutic measures are available, but relapses occur frequently.

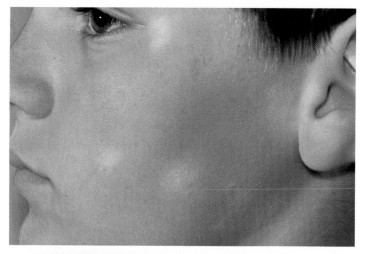

Figure 73. Pityriasis alba. Minimally scaling, round, light-colored spots on both cheeks.

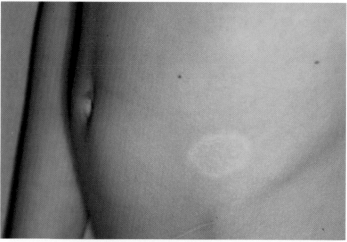

Figure 74. Pityriasis alba. Oval-shaped, minimally scaling, peripherally depigmented lesion. Left side of abdomen.

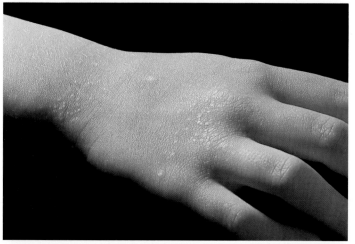

Figure 75. Juvenile papular dermatitis. Flat, grouped, whitish, and erythematous nodules on the dorsal side of metacarpophalangeal and wrist joints.

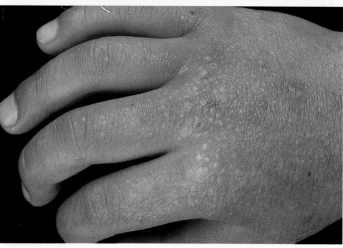

Figure 76. Juvenile papular dermatitis. Hypopigmented and erythematous nodules on the dorsum of hand and fingers.

Pityriasis Alba

This is a very superficial eczema and occurs mainly in children. It is usually visible during the summer months and is often associated with dry skin. The area of predilection is the facial skin; a suntan during the summer makes the lesions more conspicuous. The disease is harmless; its cause is unknown.

Clinical Appearance

1. A discrete white scaling is visible, occasionally only along the margin. The lesions are round, vary in size from a penny to a dollar, and are conspicuous because of their much lighter color. There is no erythema.
2. The cheeks and occasionally the forehead, neck, upper arms, abdomen, and back are involved.
3. There is no itching.

Therapy

Topical treatment is always sufficient. In many cases, no treatment is necessary. For scaling lesions, a mild ointment suffices (R.31b, c). Repigmentation occurs after approximately 4 to 6 weeks.

Juvenile Papular Dermatitis

This is a harmless eczematous disease in children that is usually disregarded. Only very attentive or worried parents will take their children to the physician's office. The cause of the disease is unknown. Treatment is not necessary. The clinical appearance of this disorder is so typical that the diagnosis can usually be made at the first glance. Children who play in the sandbox are especially at risk (sandbox dermatitis).

Clinical Appearance

1. The disorder is characterized by isolated or grouped nodules of normal skin color with no inflammatory erythema. Confluence of multiple nodules can lead to larger lesions.
2. The nodules are seen only on the knees, the elbows, and the dorsum of the hand.
3. There is no itching.

Therapy

1. In most cases, it is enough to inform the parents that the disorder is harmless.
2. Topical treatment with a bland ointment (R.31b) is usually sufficient.

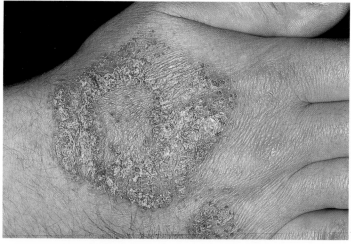

Figure 77. Nummular eczema. Round, sharply delineated, markedly scaling and crusty eczematous lesions on the dorsum of the hand.

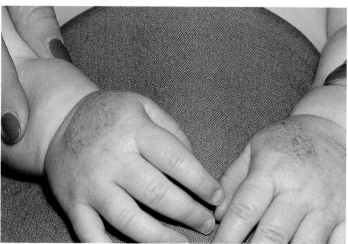

Figure 78. Nummular eczematous lesions in a patient with atopic dermatitis. Symmetric appearance of round, eczematous lesions on the dorsum of the hand.

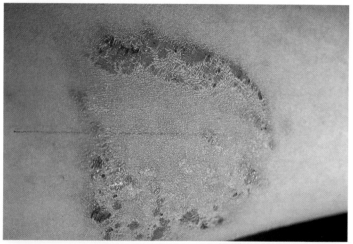

Figure 79. Nummular eczema. Erosive, papular eczematous lesion with accentuated margin.

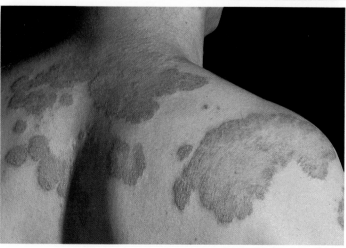

Figure 80. Nummular eczema. Extensive, partially confluent, eczematous lesions with accentuated margins.

Nummular Eczema

This condition is characterized by coin-shaped eczematous lesions that persist for prolonged periods and are very resistant to treatment. We distinguish a so-called "idiopathic" nummular eczema without a detectable cause from nummular eczematous lesions that are symptoms of other eczemas, such as atopic eczema or allergic chromate eczema. Nummular eczema in children is practically always a symptom of an atopic eczema. The cause of "idiopathic" nummular eczema is unclear. Microbial involvement has been postulated but so far has not been confirmed. The condition usually involves men of middle age or older age groups.

Clinical Appearance

1. The lesions consist of coin-shaped foci of varying sizes that are sharply delineated, round, and scaling. They are often weeping or covered with crusts and have a raised margin.
2. The extremities and trunk are involved. There may be only a few lesions, rarely 10 to 20 or more.
3. The lesions may persist for several weeks or months, frequently despite intensive topical treatment.
4. There is moderate to severe itching.
5. The skin is dry, a condition aggravated by frequent washing and bathing and by low humidity (winter, central heating).

Therapy

The prognosis depends on the type of eczema, whether the condition is part of an atopic eczema or a chromate eczema or whether it is an "idiopathic" nummular eczema that may be unexpectedly resistant to any therapy for a longer period of time.

1. The most important measure is topical treatment with corticosteroid-containing ointments (R.36b, c). Treatment should be started with a cream when weeping lesions are present. Occlusive dressings may be necessary to improve response to treatment.
2. Coal tar preparations may be used to supplement this therapy (R.37e, R.39a).
3. Severe dryness of the skin may also require treatment (see p. 139).

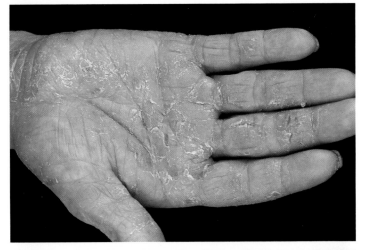

Figure 81. Chronic hyperkeratotic eczema of the palm of the hand. Typical appearance with erosions, scaling, and callus formation.

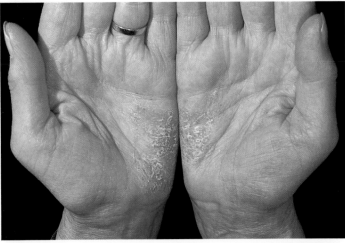

Figure 82. Chronic hyperkeratotic eczema in the palm of the hand. Lesions in early stage, not well developed.

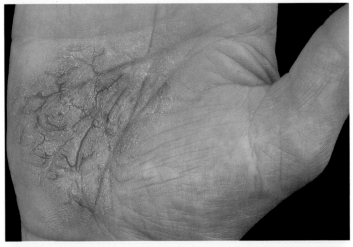

Figure 83. Chronic hyperkeratotic eczema of the palm. Callus-like keratinization with deep rhagades.

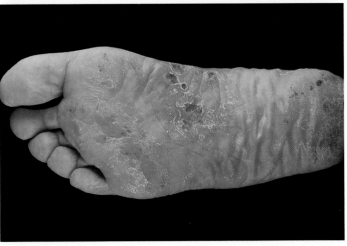

Figure 84. Chronic hyperkeratotic eczema of hands and feet. Erosions, scaling, and increased keratinization in some areas of the sole of the right foot.

Chronic Hyperkeratotic Eczema of Hands and Feet

This common disorder affects mainly middle-aged men and is characterized by inflammatory keratosis of the palms of the hands and soles of the feet. The condition can persist for many months or years and can be a significant handicap in persons who perform manual labor. The course is usually chronic and relapses are common. In most cases, no cause can be found, but in some patients, the symptoms may be due to a mycosis, a contact allergy, or an atopic dermatitis. Secondary contact sensitization occurs frequently in long-standing cases, but this usually does not play a role in the causation or maintenance of the disease.

Clinical Appearance

1. Extensive keratosis in the center or the entire skin of the palm and the soles of the feet is typical of the disease. Inflammatory changes such as erythema, groups of vesicles, erosions, and crusts predominate in some cases but can be absent in others. Painful rhagades are frequently present. They are caused by passive stretching of the thick and inelastic hyperkeratotic skin.
2. The disease involves mainly the palms and the soles of the feet. Dissemination to distant areas of the skin is rare but can occur in patients with acute eczematization.
3. Itching and pain are present in varying degrees but can be completely absent in the "dry forms" of the disease. In cases with severe hyperkeratosis, sensation and motion of hands and fingers can also be disturbed.
4. The disease runs a protracted course over many months or years. Acute flare-ups with vesicles, and so on, recur frequently without a recognizable cause.

Therapy

Treatment is a difficult and thankless task. It is typical of this disease that patients change their attending physician frequently. The goal of treatment is symptomatic improvement of the eczema and prevention of flare-ups. Flare-ups can be prevented only in those patients whose condition occurs in connection with mycoses, contact allergy, or an atopic dermatitis. Symptomatic treatment is guided by the existing symptoms.

1. The most important local measure for hyperkeratosis alone is frequent application of fatty and watery ointment bases (R.31b). If this is inadequate, ointments containing corticosteroids in conjunction with salicylic acid and tar substances, such as coal tar, may be useful, especially for chronic cases.
2. Systemic treatment is usually unnecessary. Severe flare-ups may require systemic corticosteroids in decreasing doses for a few days (R.58).

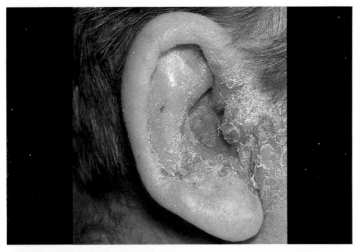

Figure 85. Bacterial ear eczema. Chronic recurrent eczema of the auditory canal and the auricle with weeping and crust formation. Marked concomitant edema of the auricle.

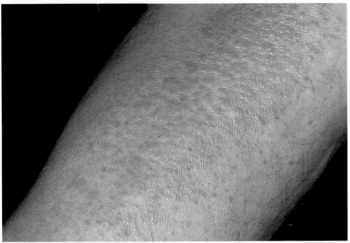

Figure 86. Lichen simplex chronicus. Severely itching eczematous nodular aggregates on the forearm.

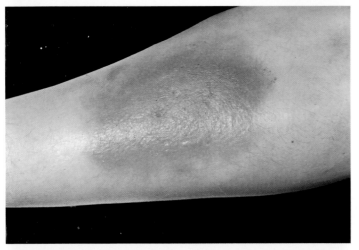

Figure 87. Lichen simplex chronicus, left lower leg. Isolated area of chronic lichenified eczema surrounded by brownish discoloration.

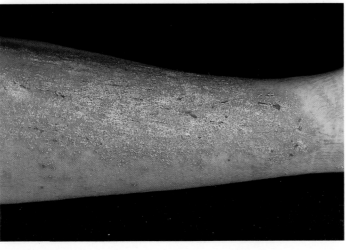

Figure 88. Lichen simplex chronicus. Chronic eczematous area that tapers off into individual nodules. The scratch marks are an indication of severe pruritus.

Bacterial Ear Eczema

This is a recurrent, crusty eczema of the ear that apparently is caused by bacterial contamination of this area. Exacerbation by generalized infection or ear infection is typical of this condition.

Clinical Appearance

1. Scaling and occasionally erythema of the external auditory canal are seen frequently. In more severe cases, weeping areas, crusts, and erosions develop. The external ear shows edematous swelling. Both ears are usually involved in varying degrees.
2. Pruritus is often agonizing.

Therapy

1. Local treatment consists of corticosteroid creams in combination with disinfectants (R.37a) and moist dressings (R.1). Corticosteroid-containing ear drops are useful for treatment of the deeper parts of the auditory canal.
2. Otologic consultation may be indicated for removal of crusts and cerumen and exclusion of otitis media.

Lichen Simplex Chronicus

This condition consists of individual chronic eczematous lesions with typical appearance. There is marked pruritus. An external cause usually cannot be found, but the patient should be evaluated for possible mechanical causes or contact allergy to exclude chronic contact eczema. Lichen simplex chronicus usually occurs in middle-aged or elderly persons, not infrequently in connection with an underlying chronic leg vein insufficiency.

Clinical Appearance

1. In typical cases, a three-zonal structure can be recognized. The outer zone shows a brownish discoloration followed by a zone of isolated eczematous nodules that coalesce toward the center into a lichenified (thickened) area. Frequently, the entire lesion has a brownish color, occasionally with interspersed depigmented areas. Scaling occurs frequently.
2. The disease has a predilection for the lower extremities, the trunk, and the back and sides of the neck.
3. The disorder is characterized by marked itching.

Therapy

Appropriate local therapy is usually sufficient. The patient should be advised not to scratch.

1. Application of corticosteroid-containing ointments (R.36c, d) to the affected areas is useful. Penetration and effectiveness of topical medication can be enhanced by the use of an occlusive wrap. Intralesional injection of a corticosteroid crystal suspension can be very effective (R.44).
2. Local application of tar (coal tar, wood tar, slate oil) in combination with corticosteroids eases itching and leads to regression of the chronic eczematization.
3. Systemic antihistamines (R.56, R.57) may be indicated for severe pruritus.

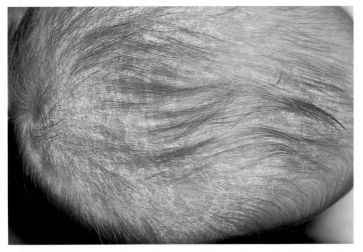

Figure 89. Atopic dermatitis. Crusta lactea. White and yellowish, slightly "fatty" scaling.

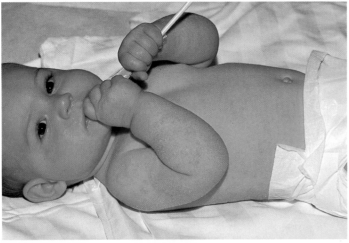

Figure 90. Atopic dermatitis. Multiple, mostly round, eczematous lesions of varying size, located on abdomen and arms.

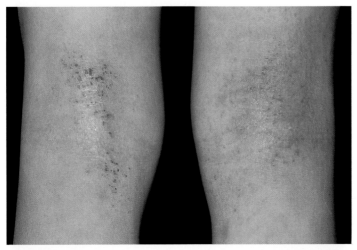

Figure 91. Atopic dermatitis. Characteristic location in the popliteal areas.

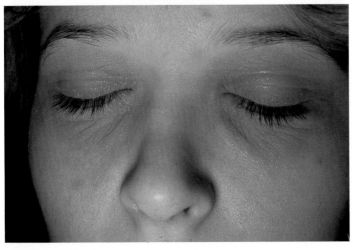

Figure 92. Atopic dermatitis. Chronic eczema of the eyelids, giving the appearance of "rings under the eyes."

Atopic Dermatitis

This skin disease is part of the atopic syndrome that also includes such disorders as bronchial asthma, allergic rhinitis, and occasionally food allergies. Atopic dermatitis is a genetically fixed disease, which means that the skin disorder or the disposition for it can be present in varying degrees during the patient's entire lifetime. The patient remains afflicted with atopic dermatitis whether skin changes are present or not. There are typical symptoms for certain age groups, such as crusta lactea in infants, flexural eczema in childhood, and finally prurigo in adults. Itching as well as other symptoms can be present in varying degrees, occasionally in an abortive stage. Pruritus is often the most agonizing symptom. Frequently, asthma worsens as the skin disorder improves and vice versa. The skin changes can appear in childhood, during puberty, or in adolescence and never recur, but in many patients the eczema persists in adulthood. Eczematous changes diminish with advancing age; atopic dermatitis is rarely seen in elderly people. The time when symptoms finally disappear, however, cannot be predicted for individual patients. In afflicted individuals, laboratory tests often show eosinophilia and elevated total IgE as well as an increase in allergen-specific IgE antibodies that can be demonstrated by RAST. The diagnosis is determined by the symptomatology and the history, not by laboratory tests, however.

Since cell-mediated immunity is disturbed in patients with atopic dermatitis, bacterial, mycotic, and viral infections are more frequent than in the general population, especially impetigo contagiosa and other pyodermas. These patients are also very susceptible to herpes simplex virus and vaccinia virus, and infections with such organisms can lead to life-threatening diseases like eczema herpeticum (see p. 71) or eczema vaccinatum.

Clinical Appearance

1. *Infantile eczema* is characterized by fine yellowish scales and very dry skin on scalp and face. The disease begins in the first few months of life, usually at the beginning of the third month.
2. *In children*, the eczema typically involves the flexor regions, such as the antecubital area, the popliteal space, and the flexor surfaces of the feet. In these areas, eczematous lesions develop with the clinical signs of chronic eczema (thickening of the skin, coarse skin markings, brownish postinflammatory pigmentation), frequently together with the symptoms of an acute eczema (erythema, nodules, weeping areas). Linear erosions and crusting are often present as a result of the patient's scratching.
3. Other eczematous lesions can be found in a widespread distribution or in patches, occasionally as nummular foci on the sides of the face, the trunk, and the extremities.
4. An important feature of atopic dermatitis is an eczema of the hand that usually manifests itself with erythema, thickening of the skin, and scaling. Occasionally, dyshidrosis is also present (see p. 29). Mild primary irritants may easily lead to exacerbation of atopic hand eczema. These changes can be severe enough to interfere with the patient's occupation, such as a baker, furrier, hairdresser, or worker in the restaurant industry, in cleaning companies, in health care, as well as in the automobile and building industry.
5. *In adolescents and adults*, prurigo nodules occur more and more and either partially or completely replace the eczematous foci.
6. Other diagnostic signs of atopic dermatitis are Hertoghe's sign (the lateral aspects of the eyebrows are thinned or absent), duplication of the fold of the lower lid with dark discoloration surrounding the eye caused by the eczema, and a fur cap shape of the hair with the margin of the hair advanced into the forehead. Frequently there is "white dermography." After strong linear pressure the initial redness does not persist for a longer period of time, as in healthy individuals, but is replaced by a reflex whiteness after a few seconds.

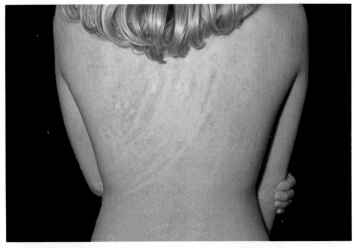

Figure 93. Atopic dermatitis. White dermographism: circumscribed vasoconstriction following linear pressure on the skin.

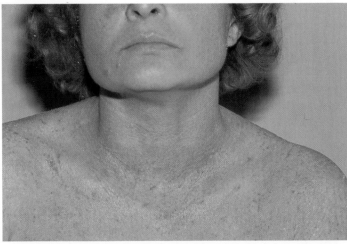

Figure 94. Atopic dermatitis. Long-standing eczema of the neck and upper chest.

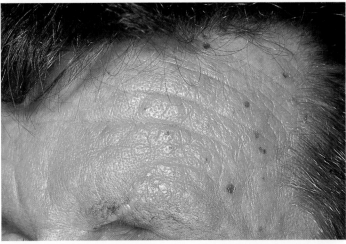

Figure 95. Atopic dermatitis. Distinct lichenification (coarser skin markings) and erosions; the lateral parts of the eyebrows are thinned (Hertoghe's sign).

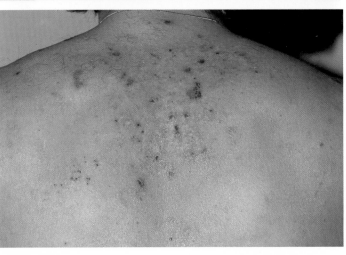

Figure 96. Atopic dermatitis; prurigo, with typical hood-shaped arrangement. The nodules have been scratched open. Areas of depigmentation and hyperpigmentation.

7. Patients with atopic dermatitis suffer from dry skin that is worse during the winter months.
8. Pruritus is practically always present and can be quite annoying. This leads to constant scratching even during sleep. The patient sleeps poorly and is often tired during the day, which exaggerates the itching. There is intolerance to sheep's wool, which causes severe itching.
9. Emotional factors often play an important role. Many patients with atopic dermatitis have above average intelligence. On the outside they appear calm but often suffer from fear, frustrations, insecurity, and aggression. Emotional problems can be caused by childhood eczema but may also be due to an unconscious resentment of and lack of affection by the mother.

Therapy

Since most patients with atopic dermatitis suffer considerably from their eczema and pruritus, they cooperate quite well with treatment.

General

1. Vacation at the sea or in the mountains usually results in significant but temporary improvement.
2. Breastfeeding appears to lessen manifestation of the disease in patients with a disposition to infantile eczema. The often-recommended diet changes (buttermilk, sauerkraut, and many others) have no effect on the eczema. In some patients, citrus fruits can cause exacerbation of the disease. Allergies to certain foods are more frequent than in the general population. This, however, may not aggravate the eczema. Clinical symptoms of food allergies consist of diarrhea, vomiting, and colic with increased intestinal sounds.

Systemic

Systemic drug therapy is not without problems, because it must be given over a long period of time and this often increases side effects and habit formation.

1. Severe pruritus may require the use of antihistamines (R.56, R.57). Those with a sedative component may be preferable because they enable the patients, even children, to get a good night's sleep. With long-term use, tachyphylaxis may reduce effectiveness of the drug, and increasingly higher doses may be necessary.
2. Systemic corticosteroids should be avoided if possible. They usually produce prompt improvement, but symptoms recur when the drug is discontinued, and there is risk of drug dependence.

External

1. It is important from a therapeutic as well as a prophylactic point of view to treat dry skin with frequent applications of a hydrophilic ointment without active medication (R. 31). Creams are usually insufficient. Fatty externa should not be applied too thickly, otherwise they can aggravate the skin condition.
2. For acute eczematous lesions, moist compresses are helpful, or corticosteroid lotions (emulsion type) can be used for several days.
3. For chronic eczemas, interval therapy (see p. 226) with corticosteroid-containing ointments (R.36) and tar preparations (R.37d, e) are helpful. In children, only weak corticosteroids (R.36a) should be used topically.
4. A full bath with the addition of bath oil or a bath oil with tar preparation is indicated every day or every second day. To avoid desiccation of the skin, an ointment without active medication should be applied to the moist skin immediately after the bath.
5. For adolescents and adults, a sauna bath two or three times weekly is beneficial.
6. Sun bathing or artificial UV radiation produces significant improvement in many patients.

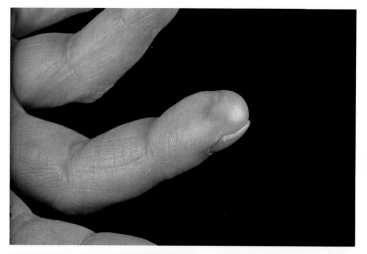

Figure 97. Second degree frostbite: Bulla on the fingertip with surrounding erythema.

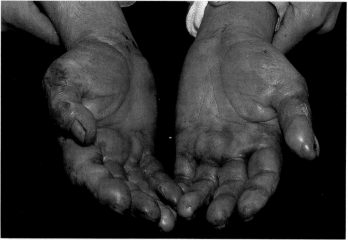

Figure 98. Second degree frostbite: Erosions, bullae, and livid discoloration of the fingers.

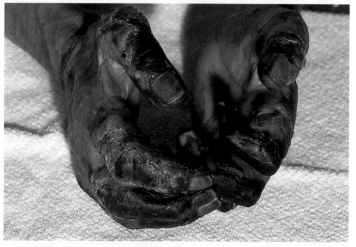

Figure 99. Sequelae of second-degree frostbite under treatment.

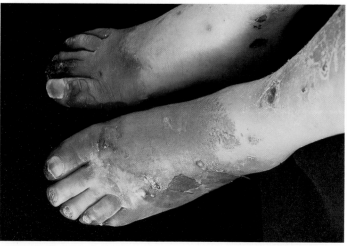

Figure 100. Third-degree frostbite of the foot. Erythema, formation of bullae, desquamation of the epidermis, and necrosis of the distal phalanges with mummification.

Frostbite

Frostbite is sudden, circumscribed tissue damage that occurs in temperatures below the freezing point. Ears, nose, cheeks, hands, and feet are affected most frequently. Frostbite is seen most often in winter sports, not infrequently in conjunction with increased alcohol consumption. It can also occur with sudden cold spells in persons wearing inadequate clothing (motorcyclists). Various degrees of tissue damage similar to that caused by burns can be identified. Pathogenetic factors include damage to the blood supply, direct cold injury to the cells, and possibly injury due to ice crystal formation in the tissues.

Clinical Appearance

First Degree Frostbite

During cold exposure, the skin of the involved areas is white and much colder than the surrounding skin. Following rewarming, edematous swelling occurs that often itches markedly. This swelling continues to increase, initially due to the liberation of substances that mediate inflammation, and then slowly disappears over a period of several days without sequelae.

Second Degree Frostbite

The skin is waxy and pale. After rewarming, subepidermal blisters appear, similar to those seen in burns. These blisters are very painful and can occasionally be hemorrhagic.

Third Degree Frostbite

After third degree frostbite, the damaged skin remains white following rewarming and sensation is absent. The necrotic area develops a blue-black color, and the hardened tissue is slowly demarcated from the surrounding healthy tissue. Development of wet gangrene with the risk of bacterial sepsis is a serious complication. It is often surprising that only a relatively small defect results after demarcation, despite extensive tissue damage initially. Pain and paresthesias in the affected areas can persist for many years and disable the patient.

Therapy

1. It is important to rewarm the affected tissue areas as soon as possible. Rewarming should be done gradually, preferably in a bath of cold tap water that is heated slowly (in approximately 1 1/2 hours) to 40° C.
2. The patient should be given warm drinks (but no alcohol) to raise his or her body temperature, followed by rheologically active medications such as Pentoxifyllin, Naftidrofuryl, Buflomedil, and prostaglandin E. Tetanus prophylaxis is also important.
3. Patients with severe undercooling must be transported carefully. Vasodilating drugs should be administered with great caution. The sudden return of cold peripheral blood will lower the core temperature of the body even more, with the risk of respiratory and cardiac arrest and irreversible CNS damage.
4. Sympathetic blocking by continuous peridural anesthesia is reported to be very effective if done as soon as possible.
5. Frostbite should be treated open and dry. Under no circumstances should wet dressings or ointments be used (danger of wet gangrene). Interdigital spaces are kept dry by insertion of small gauze strips. The involved skin is painted with disinfectant dyes (R.14, R.17) and powdered (R.12).
6. The tissue regenerates extremely well after frostbite, and surgical procedures such as excision of necroses and amputations should be delayed as long as possible. Patience is the most important therapeutic principle.

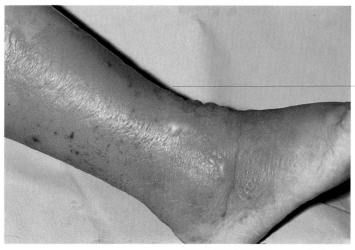

Figure 101. Erysipelas. Acute stage with erythema, edema, and blistering.

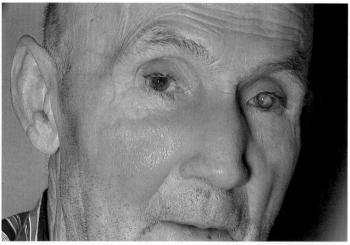

Figure 102. Erysipelas of the face. Sharply delineated, unilateral erythema involving cheek and nose.

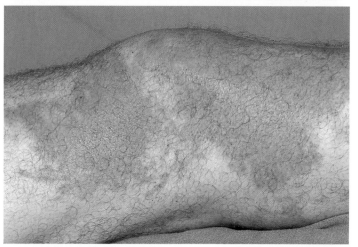

Figure 103. Erysipelas. Widespread erythema with striped margins corresponding to the inflammation that advances along the lymph vessels.

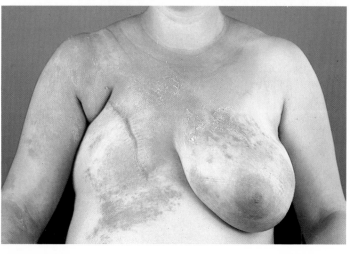

Figure 104. Erysipelas following mastectomy. Extensive involvement including the right arm, caused by postoperative lymphatic stasis.

Erysipelas

Erysipelas is a dermal streptococcal infection that progresses along the superficial lymphatics. The disease involves mainly older adults. Recurrent flare-ups with subsequent chronic persistent lymphedema are possible (see p. 97). "Erysipeloid" thrombophlebitis can produce similar symptoms but always involves both lower legs without enlargement of lymph nodes and without generalized symptoms. The erythema stops below the knees, like knee-length stockings.

Clinical Appearance

1. The disease is characterized by intense redness with acute onset. The erythema is irregular and has extensions like "fiery tongues" (along the lymph vessels).
2. The disorder is usually unilateral, but bilateral involvement is seen occasionally, especially in the face.
3. Lower legs and face are affected most frequently.
4. The skin symptoms are accompanied by chills, fever, and swelling of the regional lymph nodes.
5. Local complications are vesiculations, hemorrhagic infarction, ulceration, and necrosis of the inflamed area. Severe sepsis occurs as a rare complication.
6. Frequent recurrences can occasionally cause occlusion of the lymph vessels, with subsequent edema that can be extremely severe in some cases (elephantiasis) (see p. 97).

Therapy

Systemic antibiotic therapy is the most important part of treatment, but general measures and topical treatment are also necessary.

General

1. Bedrest is recommended.
2. Elevation of the involved extremity is helpful to reduce swelling and pain.

Systemic

1. Antibiotic therapy takes precedence. Penicillin (R.45) is the drug of choice, either orally or more effectively by intramuscular administration. Erythromycin (R.49) or tetracyclines (R.47) are also effective and can be used in patients with hypersensitivity to penicillin.
2. Analgesics, such as acetylsalicylic acid or paracetamol are sometimes required.
3. In patients with frequent recurrences of erysipelas, prophylaxis with long-term antibiotic therapy (e.g., 1.2 million units benzathine benzyl penicillin intramuscularly, once every 4 weeks) may be necessary for at least several months.

External

Local therapy depends on the extent of the skin involvement. As long as only redness is present, local therapy can be omitted.

1. Moist dressings (R.1, R.2) are soothing and are always helpful.
2. Antibiotic ointments are widely used, but their effectiveness is questionable.
3. Skin lesions, such as small wounds, rhagades, interdigital mycosis, or eczema of the ear, which can serve as entry portals for organisms, should be treated with appropriate local therapy to prevent recurrence.

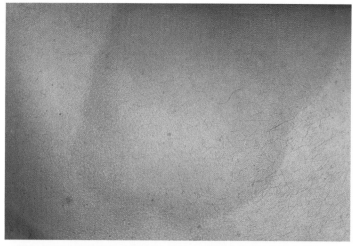

Figure 105. Erythema chronicum migrans. Round or polycyclical erythema with distinct margins.

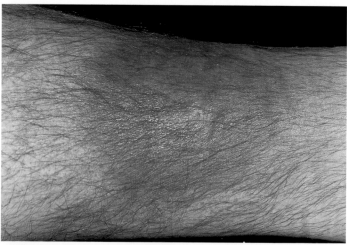

Figure 106. Hemorrhagic erythema chronicum migrans. Purpuric round erythema without distinct margins.

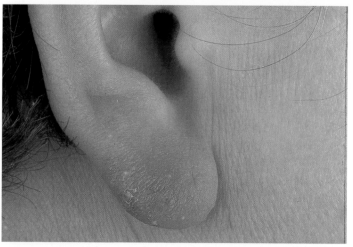

Figure 107. Lymphocytoma. Burgundy to bluish-red colored tumor-like infiltrate of the right earlobe.

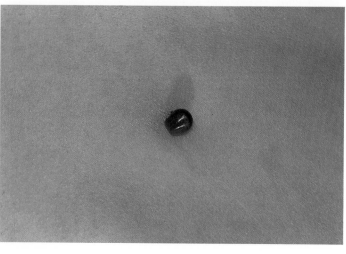

Figure 108. Wood tick, *Ixodes ricinus*, with enlarged abdomen from sucking blood.

Erythema Chronicum Migrans and Other Skin Disorders Transmitted by Ticks

Erythema chronicum migrans and acrodermatitis chronica atrophicans are superficial infectious diseases of the skin. They are caused by Borrelia burgdorferi *and possibly other spirochetes transmitted by* Ixodes ricinus *in Europe and by* I. scapularis, pacificus, *and* dammini *in the United States. The ticks usually get into the skin when the patient walks through brush. Lymphocytoma can also be transmitted by ticks, but there can be other causes of the disease.*

Erythema Chronicum Migrans

Clinical Appearance

1. Erythema chronicum migrans is a slowly enlarging round erythema with an accentuated margin. Hemorrhagic changes in the lesion can obliterate the accentuated margin.
2. The lesion enlarges slowly over a period of several weeks. Multiple foci are rare.
3. The disorder involves not only the areas of the body directly exposed to the ticks but also other parts of the body covered by clothing because the tick can move under the clothing.
4. Erythema chronicum migrans can be a symptom of Lyme disease, which is characterized by mono- or polyarticular arthritis, especially of the large joints, and neurologic symptoms such as meningitis, encephalitis, radicular neuritis, and occasionally there can be cardiac involvement.

Therapy

Systemic antibiotic therapy is the treatment of choice. Systemic tetracyclines (R.47) (orally for 2 weeks), penicillin (R.45), or erythromycin (R.49) effect rapid disappearance of the lesions. Local therapy is not necessary.

Acrodermatitis Chronica Atrophicans

This disease occurs less frequently than erythema chronicum migrans, but it is transmitted in the same manner. Clinical symptoms vary from those of erythema chronicum migrans.

Clinical Appearance

1. Initial symptoms develop slowly and include erythema and swelling of large areas of the skin, frequently of an entire extremity.
2. The disease eventually leads to atrophy of the skin. The skin is thin and can be folded easily into fine folds. Underlying blood vessels, especially veins, can be seen easily through the skin.

Therapy

Treatment is the same as for erythema chronicum migrans but must be given over a period of several weeks. The skin atrophy is permanent and is not altered by treatment.

Lymphocytoma

Clinical Appearance

1. This disease occurs as solitary, very rarely as disseminated multiple, bluish-red, round or oval tumors up to 3 cm in size. It can also occur in the center of erythema chronicum migrans at the site of the tick bite.
2. The most frequent localization is in the face, especially the earlobe and tip of the nose. Scrotum and mamillae can also be affected.
3. There are no subjective complaints.

Therapy

The same as for erythema chronicum migrans.

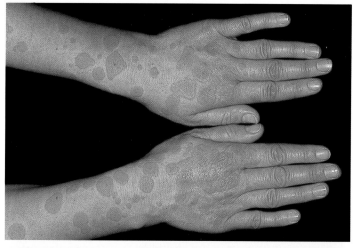

Figure 109. Erythema multiforme on both arms. Typical raised erythematous, up to penny-size lesions with central dusky discoloration caused by stasis.

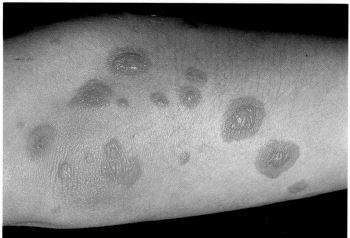

Figure 110. Erythema multiforme. Blister formation in the center of the lesions.

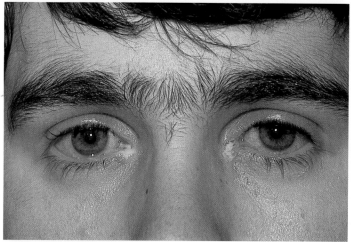

Figure 111. Erythema multiforme. Involvement of the eyes as indicated by conjunctival injection and purulent secretion into the conjunctival sac.

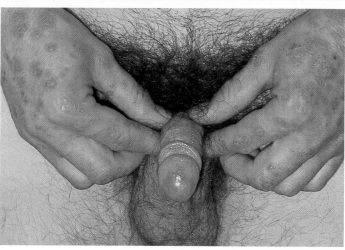

Figure 112. Erythema multiforme. Typical lesions on the dorsum of both hands as well as involvement of the genitals.

Erythema Multiforme

Erythema multiforme is a special form of hypersensitivity reaction of the skin to various causative agents. In many cases, these agents are not identifiable; in others, erythema multiforme may accompany or follow bacterial or viral infection. Less commonly, it can be started by drugs, x-rays, or a sarcoidosis. The disorder usually affects young people and heals within 3 to 6 weeks, depending on initial involvement. It is important to identify the causative agents or diseases (e.g., recurrent herpes simplex or Mycoplasma pneumoniae).

Clinical Appearance

1. The disease is characterized by circinate or iris-shaped, concentric, penny-sized foci with a tendency to form blisters. Involvement is often symmetric. Old and new lesions can be found side by side.
2. Involvement of the dorsum of the hand and the forearm is typical; occasionally, the palms and soles of both feet are affected. Widespread involvement of the entire skin is also possible.
3. The mucous membranes adjacent to the skin can be involved, especially when the disease is widespread. The conjunctivae are reddened ("tearful eyes"). In some patients, involvement of the oral mucous membranes is present, with hemorrhagic crusts on the lips. Stomatitis frequently presents itself in the anterior parts of the oral mucosa with erosions, ulcerations, and fibrinous coatings. The patients often have an unpleasant mouth odor. The genital mucous membranes can also be affected.
4. Moderate to marked pruritus is usually present.
5. In the beginning, the patient often complains of malaise, joint pain, and fever.

Therapy

Systemic

1. In severe cases (typus major with mucous membrane involvement, Stevens-Johnson syndrome), short-term systemic corticosteroid treatment is indicated. For example, high doses of prednisolone or another corticosteroid for 3 days, followed by gradual reduction of the dose as clinical symptoms improve.
2. Analgesics may be necessary for severe stomatitis.
3. For severe pruritus, oral antihistamines (R.56, R.57) may be necessary for several days.

External

1. Local therapy is not necessary for mild involvement without bullae.
2. Bullae should be treated by local disinfection (R.17) and evacuation; otherwise a shake lotion (R.20a, c) is sufficient.
3. Stomatitis may require frequent mouthwash with lukewarm water, possibly with the addition of antiseptics (e.g., 0.1 to 0.3% H_2O_2 solution = 1 teaspoon of 3% H_2O_2 solution in one glass of water.)
4. Topical application of corticosteroids does not influence the disease significantly.

General

Bedrest is recommended. Patients with severe and extensive involvement of the mucous membranes should have a liquid or soft diet. Hospitalization may be necessary for severe cases.

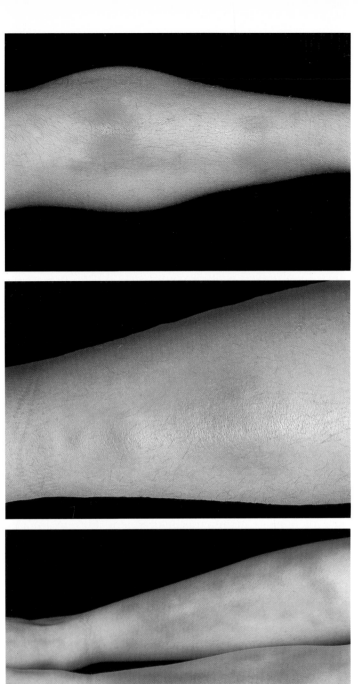

Figure 113. Erythema nodosum. Painful nodular infiltrates in the pretibial area.

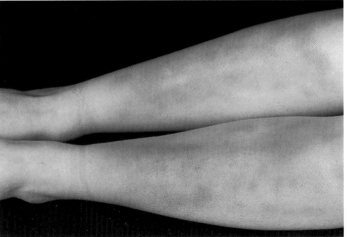

Figure 114. Erythema nodosum. Tight, shiny skin over an acute inflammatory infiltrate.

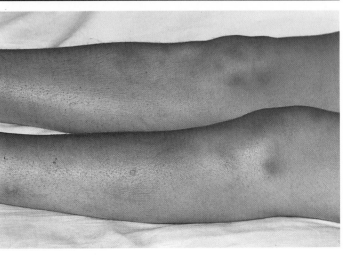

Figure 115. Erythema nodosum contusiforme. Brownish discoloration of infiltrates resembling hematomas.

Figure 116. Erythema nodosum. Multiple nodular lesions on both lower legs and knees.

Erythema Nodosum

Erythema nodosum is a special form of hypersensitivity reaction of the skin that can be due to a variety of factors. It may accompany bacterial or viral infections, such as angina tonsillaris, pharyngitis, yersiniosis, BCG vaccination, or tuberculosis. It can also be associated with sarcoidosis (Löfgren's syndrome), Crohn's disease, or ulcerative colitis, or it can be induced by drugs (e.g., sulfonamides, phenacetin, penicillin). In most patients, however, an internal or external cause cannot be identified. The disease affects mainly young women; erythema nodosum rarely occurs in old age.

Clinical Appearance

1. The typical eruption consists of painful nodular infiltrates on the lower legs, especially in the pretibial area. They are reddened and can develop a hematoma-like brown or green discoloration after they have been present for some time (contusiform appearance).
2. The lesions are painful to a point where even the weight of the quilt can cause pain.
3. Multiple lesions are usually present.
4. Erythema nodosum occurs on the extensor sides of the lower legs and occasionally on the thighs. It rarely affects other parts of the body.
5. Constitutional symptoms consist of joint pains (knee and ankle joints, occasionally other joints), initially also fever, malaise, and headaches.
6. Isolated attacks occur frequently and resolve completely within a few weeks. New infiltrates often occur over longer time periods; erythema nodosum can last for several months.

Therapy

After possible causative diseases have been excluded or treated, therapy of the skin condition is usually symptomatic.

1. The most important local measure is bedrest with elevation of the legs. A tunnel can minimize pain from pressure of the quilt.
2. Corticosteroid ointments (R.36c) can be used with an occlusive foil, but pathologic changes are often found in a deep cutaneous location and topical therapy usually cannot reach the lesions. Cooling with moist dressings often has a soothing effect.
3. Nonsteroidal anti-inflammatory agents such as acetylsalicylic acid are occasionally helpful.
4. Systemic corticosteroid therapy with medium doses (see p. 238) should be used only in severe cases. Of course, corticosteroids should not be given when infection is present.

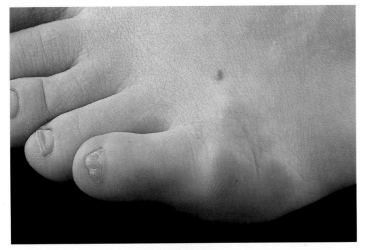

Figure 117. Chilblains. Bluish-red, painful infiltrate with pruritus.

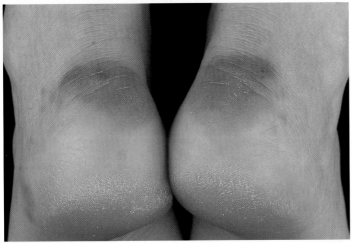

Figure 118. Chilblains. Symmetric, bluish-red infiltrates in areas exposed to cold.

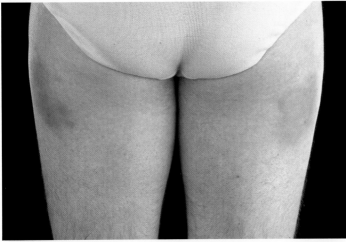

Figure 119. Chilblains can develop in areas covered by tight clothing (jeans). Characteristic location on the outside of both thighs in young women; frequently caused by bicycling and horseback riding (cold panniculitis).

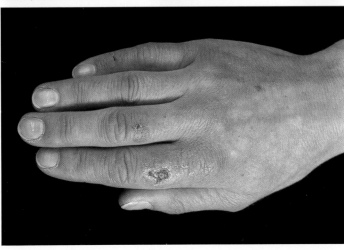

Figure 120. Chilblains with ulcerations (rare).

Chilblain, Pernio

Chilblains are circumscribed inflammatory changes that occur in predisposed patients after exposure to moderate cold. Genetic disposition and functional disturbance of the blood supply often exist with acrocyanosis or cold clammy fingers and toes. Other factors such as diet, clothing, and atmospheric humidity may also play a role. Chilblains usually occur in damp, cold weather. They are rare in countries with very cold and dry winters because the dry air conducts temperature poorly and people usually wear appropriate clothing. Girls and young women are predominantly affected.

Nodular infiltrates, especially on the lateral and posterolateral aspects of the thighs are called cold panniculitis. They are frequently seen in young women after horseback riding or bicycling. In infants, these changes often develop on the cheeks as a reaction to cold exposure following long rides in a baby carriage.

Clinical Appearance

1. Bluish-red circumscribed nodular swellings are typical. In severe cases or with continued exposure to cold, blister formation and ulceration can occur.
2. Areas of predilection are the dorsal aspects of fingers and toes, the heels, and the lower legs. The hips can be involved when tight clothing is worn.
3. Rewarming leads to marked itching and occasionally severe pain.

Therapy

After exposure to cold has ceased, the pathologic changes heal spontaneously within 7 to 14 days. Prophylactic measures must be taken to prevent recurrent attacks. The patient must be advised to wear dry, well-insulated shoes and to avoid tight-fitting clothes. Athletic activities are important for vascular training.

Systemic

Vasodilating drugs enhance blood supply (Nifedipine). Antihistamines (R.56) are recommended for severe itching.

External

Topical therapy is of little value. In some patients, baths with addition of substances to induce hyperemia, such as benzylnicotinate, salicylamide, and other substances that stimulate the skin may be effective. For severe inflammation, a short course of corticosteroids (R.36b) may be indicated.

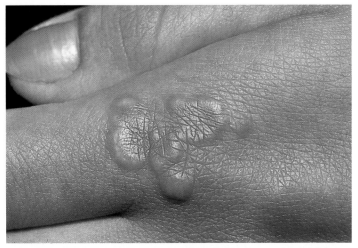

Figure 121. Granuloma annulare. Lesion with scalloped borders and small nodules in the margin.

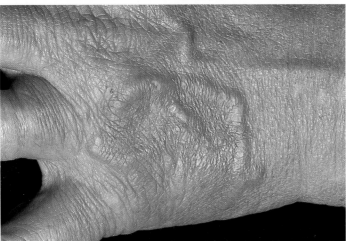

Figure 122. Granuloma annulare. Typical lesion over the knuckles with mild pitting at the center.

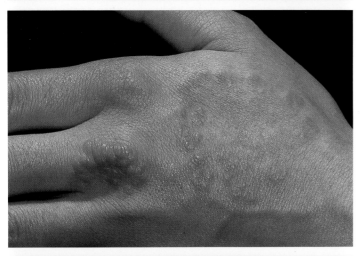

Figure 123. Granuloma annulare. Distinct raised margin composed of multiple small nodules.

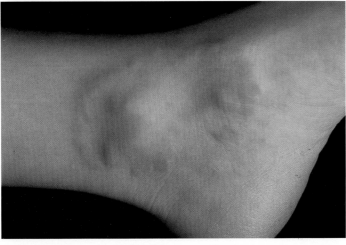

Figure 124. Granuloma annulare. The malleolar region is frequently involved, brownish discoloration of the affected area.

Granuloma Annulare, Necrobiosis Lipoidica

Granuloma Annulare

This chronic inflammatory disease mainly affects children but can also affect adults. Its cause is unknown. In adults, it is occasionally associated with diabetes mellitus. A related disorder, necrobiosis lipoidica, is more often associated with diabetes mellitus. Granuloma annulare can exist for months, or even years, and then involute spontaneously. The lesions consist of individual nodules that can be shown histologically. If in doubt, the diagnosis can be confirmed microscopically (characteristic histologic appearance).

Clinical Appearance

1. Usually there are several annular lesions with a marginal rim of flesh-colored to erythematous, slightly raised nodules. Initially, the center of the lesion is skin colored, later changing to a dusky to brownish-red color. In older lesions, the nodular rim may not be distinctly visible. These lesions can appear as sharply delineated, round, persistent, pale or dusky-brown discolorations. The epidermis is always unchanged.
2. Areas of predilection are the dorsal surfaces of the finger and toe joints, but granuloma annulare can also appear in other parts of the body, especially the extremities and trunk.
3. Usually, there are no subjective symptoms except for occasional mild itching.

Therapy

The results of treatment are not satisfactory. In patients with diabetes, the blood sugar must be kept within normal limits.

1. These patients are often worried by the persistent and slowly spreading eruptions and should be informed about the harmless nature of their disease.
2. Corticosteroid ointments (R.36c) under an occlusive foil are sometimes effective.
3. Intralesional injection of a corticosteroid crystal suspension (R.44) is often helpful.
4. Occasionally, the lesions disappear spontaneously or after biopsy.

Necrobiosis Lipoidica

Necrobiosis lipoidica affects mainly young and middle-aged adults. Its cause is unknown. It frequently occurs in diabetics, but a manifest or latent diabetes or a diabetic disposition cannot be found in all patients. Women are affected three times more often than are men. The lesions develop and spread slowly over a period of many years.

Clinical Appearance

1. Typical lesions are dusky-red to light brown flat nodules and later plaques that develop central atrophy with yellow discoloration and enlarged blood vessels. In approximately 25 percent of all patients, the granuloma ulcerates. There may be individual or multiple foci.
2. Most frequently, the lesions are located on the anterior aspect of the lower leg.
3. The lesions are usually not painful, even those with ulcers.

Therapy

1. Confirmation or exclusion of diabetes mellitus is important. An existing diabetes mellitus must be brought under optimal control, but even this does not regularly improve necrobiosis lipoidica.
2. Intralesional injections of a corticosteroid crystal suspension either with a hypodermic needle or Dermo-jet can improve the symptoms.

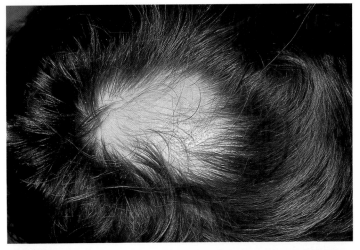

Figure 125. Alopecia areata. Circumscribed round area of baldness without visible inflammatory changes.

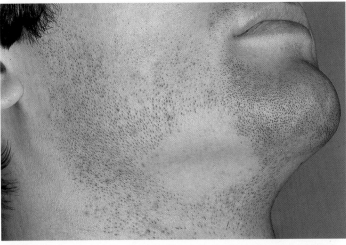

Figure 126. Alopecia areata. Circumscribed round area of baldness in the region of the beard.

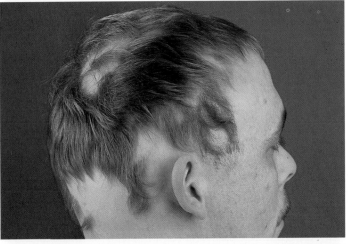

Figure 127. Alopecia areata. Multiple, partly coalescing alopecia lesions of varying sizes.

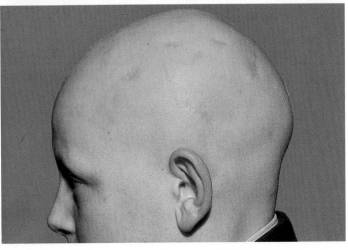

Figure 128. Alopecia areata totalis with absence of eyelids and eyelashes. The pitted atrophic areas were caused by subcutaneous injections of a corticosteroid crystal suspension.

Diseases of the Hair

Alopecia Areata

This disease frequently appears in recurring attacks and affects men as often as it does women. It often manifests itself in childhood; it rarely begins after age 40. The cause of the disease is unknown. Different factors, such as genetic disposition or immunologic mechanisms, seem to play a role. In individual cases, emotional stress (accidents, examinations, mourning) can be identified as predisposing causes. Sometimes the patient suffers also from atopic dermatitis (see p. 47) or from vitiligo (see p. 101). The course of the disease varies. Complete recovery can take place after a few weeks, but in extreme cases, there can be total and permanent loss of all body hair.

Clinical Appearance

1. Complete loss of hair in round patches without signs of pathologic changes in the underlying skin, such as scaling, inflammation, or atrophy, are characteristic. At first, the regrowing hairs are thin and without pigment (downy hair).
2. Alopecia areata affects mainly the scalp, but the lesions can occur in other hairy regions of the body, especially eyebrows and bearded areas. In severe cases (alopecia universalis), there is loss of all body hair.
3. Other symptoms, such as itching, are absent.

Therapy

Treatment of alopecia areata is still unsatisfactory. The course of the disease is unpredictable, and many "cures" following a specific treatment must be regarded as spontaneous recoveries.

Patients should be informed about the nature of the disease to keep them from seeking help through "mystic" or very expensive and questionable treatments.

Systemic

1. Corticosteroids in doses of 20 to 50 mg prednisolone produce new hair growth, but the effect is not lasting. The undesirable side effects of corticosteroids far outweigh their therapeutic benefits for this disease. They are indicated only in exceptional cases.
2. Sulfur-containing amino acids, vitamins, trace elements, especially zinc, have been recommended, but their effectiveness has not been confirmed.
3. Photochemotherapy (PUVA) is helpful in some patients.

Topical

1. Creation of an allergic contact dermatitis with Diphencyprone appears promising. This procedure is in the experimental stage and cannot be recommended for general use at this time.
2. Intralesional injection of corticosteroid crystal suspension can be tried for lesions of alopecia areata. (Caution: may produce atrophy.)
3. Hyperemia-producing substances can cause hair to grow occasionally in a patient. This can also be achieved by producing a nonantigenic irritant dermatitis with anthralin.
4. In patients with extensive scalp involvement, a wig may be helpful.
5. Surgical procedures (hair transplants) are not advisable because of the unpredictable nature of the disease.

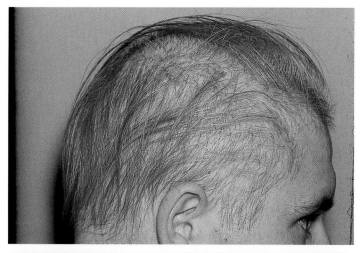

Figure 129. Diffuse alopecia following thallium poisoning.

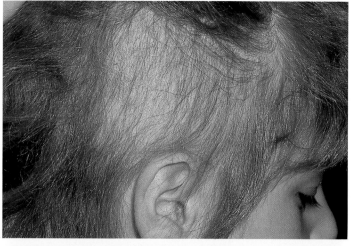

Figure 130. Trichotillomania. Habitual pulling out of hair in a circumscribed area.

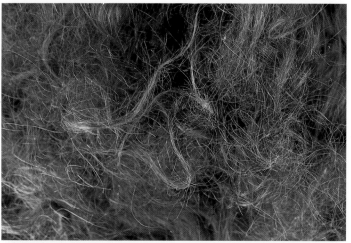

Figure 131. Toxic damage to the hair caused by the liquid used for cold waves. The hair is severely matted and cannot be combed.

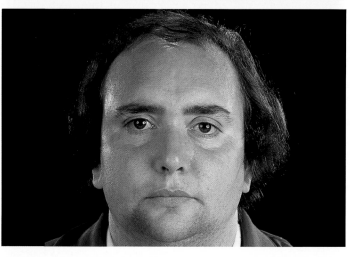

Figure 132. Hirsutism. Androgenic alopecia and beard development in a 28-year-old woman.

Diffuse Alopecia

In women, alopecia, especially androgenetic alopecia of the male type, is usually a sign of hormonal disturbance (androgen-producing tumors). In men, early onset and rapid progression can lead to significant cosmetic impairment, especially in patients with a vulnerable emotional structure. There may be transient diffuse alopecias after acute generalized disorders, infectious diseases, operations, and pregnancy and delivery. They can be due to medications, such as cytostatic and anticoagulant drugs, thyrostatic drugs, or intoxication (e.g., thallium).

Clinical Appearance

1. Alopecia of the male type begins with a receding hairline, followed by a circumscribed bald area on the occiput (tonsure); the area where the hair is parted becomes thinner. Eventually only a seam of hair remains over the ears and the occiput.
2. In contrast to this, androgenetic alopecia of the female type initially shows thinning of the hair in the entire parietal area, whereas the hairline remains unchanged.
3. In alopecia caused by toxicity, the entire scalp is evenly affected.

Therapy

Of primary importance for the management of androgenetic alopecia in women is the evaluation of the underlying hormonal disorder and its treatment. In men, appropriate treatment is determined largely by the psychic structure of the patient. In transient diffuse alopecia, identification of the causative agent is important. A specific therapy is not necessary. Complete regrowth will occur.

Systemic

Androgenetic alopecia in women requires antiandrogen therapy with cyproterone acetate. Before menopause this is done in combination with estrogen as a contraceptive.

External

1. Estrogen-containing hair lotion in combination with corticosteroids (R.18) may be recommended (only in women).
2. Antiseborrheic shampoos (R.10) for oily, scaling scalp improve the cosmetic appearance.
3. Preliminary studies have shown minoxidil tincture to be effective for androgenetic alopecia in men.
4. Other topical remedies, trace elements, vitamins, or scalp massage are not successful. Hair transplants and other plastic surgical procedures are expensive and rarely lead to acceptable results. It is more sensible to prescribe a wig.

Trichotillomania

This disorder is characterized by habitual pulling out of hair and is seen mostly in children. It is usually caused by emotional problems (familial conflict situations, school stress); a serious psychiatric disease is rarely found. Constant pulling of the hair gradually leads to a bald area with hair of varying lengths. Regrowth of hair is normal. The hair of the scalp and less frequently the eyebrows and eyelashes are the sites usually involved.

Therapy

Patient and parents should be informed about the nature of the disorder. The basic emotional problems should be solved.

External Damage to the Hair

These disorders are usually caused by cosmetic fashions, such as excessive combing and brushing; excessive washing, dyeing, or bleaching; permanent waves or straightening of curly hair; and so forth.

Clinical Appearance

Appearance depends on the causative factors and may include increased fragility, split hairs, and even matted, unmanageable hair.

Therapy

The damage is usually limited to the hair shaft. Removal of the causative factors will lead to regrowth of healthy, normal hair in most cases.

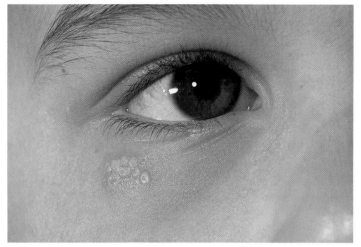

Figure 133. Recurrent herpes simplex. Grouped, pitted vesicles on inflammatory erythema, partly converted into pustules.

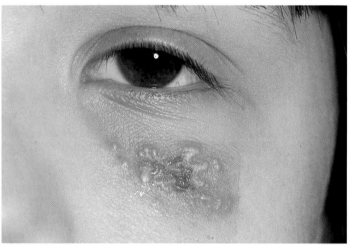

Figure 134. Herpes simplex. Grouped vesicles and pustules with crust formation.

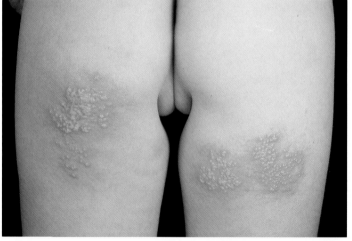

Figure 135. Herpes simplex multilocularis. Widespread herpes simplex lesions that always recur at the same site.

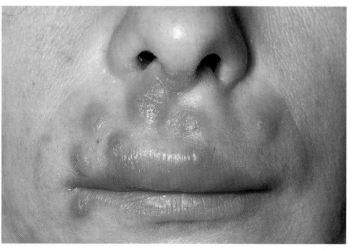

Figure 136. Recurrent herpes simplex of the lip region. The lesions extend to the nostrils.

Herpes Simplex

Diseases caused by herpes simplex virus are among the most frequent infectious diseases of the skin. Primary and secondary or recurrent infections vary in their clinical appearance and their course. Primary infections usually occur during childhood and are often completely asymptomatic. Recurrences develop in some patients in intervals of a few weeks and are therefore seen much more frequently by the practicing physician. Two serotypes of the herpes simplex virus (HSV) can be distinguished. As a rule, HSV-I is responsible for herpes lesions in most areas of the body, except genital and anal lesions, which are caused by HSV-II. The herpes virus is transmitted by direct contact or by droplet infection. Primary and secondary eruptions remain contagious for approximately 4 days. Recurrences are caused by reactivation of latent organisms that have remained in the body after a primary infection. Reactivation can be triggered by menses, trauma, UV radiation, or febrile infections, as such symptoms as flu blisters or fever blisters indicate. The incidence of recurrent attacks varies considerably between different patients; they become less frequent with advancing age.

A severe form of herpes simplex infection occurs in patients with atopic dermatitis, so-called eczema herpeticum. These patients have a deficiency of cell-mediated immunity, and the herpes virus spreads very rapidly over large areas of the skin. Primary infections of this disease are also more severe than recurrent manifestations.

Clinical Appearance

Primary Manifestations

1. Primary infection with herpes simplex virus manifests itself as acute gingivostomatitis, vulvovaginitis or balanitis, and urethritis. The clinical manifestations consist of densely grouped blisters, erosions, and purulent, malodorous crusts. Skin eruptions, as in widespread recurrent herpes simplex, are also possible.
2. Hypersensitivity and pain in the affected area shortly before eruption of the lesion are the earliest symptoms.
3. The lesions are quite painful and are accompanied by swelling of the regional lymph nodes. There can be high fever, especially with extensive involvement of the oral mucosa.

Recurrent Manifestations

1. The patients often complain of a feeling of tension and itching in the affected area before the eruptions appear.
2. The typical eruption consists of grouped, centrally pitted, clear vesicles that later change into pustules. After a short time, erosions with polycyclic borders develop, often covered with hemorrhagic fibrinous, occasionally purulent, crusts.
3. The most frequently involved site is the face, especially lips and nares. The genital region may also be involved: in women, the vulva; in men, the glans penis and the prepuce (transmission through intercourse). Herpes simplex infections can appear in any region of the body; recurrent attacks usually occur at the previously involved site.
4. The lesions are often accompanied by a painful swelling of the lymph nodes. With recurrent attacks, the course of the disease is much less severe than it is with primary infections.
5. Involvement of the eye, with the development of herpes keratitis, is a serious complication that can lead to scarring and impaired vision. Ophthalmologic consultation is necessary in these cases. Occasionally, herpes simplex infection can be complicated by erythema multiforme (see p. 57).
6. Herpes simplex of the birth canal is an indication for cesarean section to avoid infection of the child. (Herpes sepsis of the newborn has a high mortality rate.)

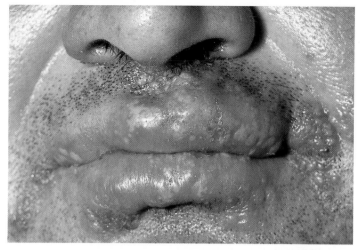

Figure 137. Recurrent herpes simplex. Multiple individual lesions involving the lips.

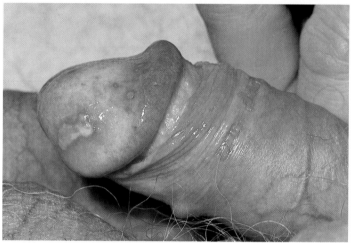

Figure 138. Genital herpes simplex. Round or polycyclic (through confluence of lesions) erosions on glans penis and prepuce that are coated with fibrin.

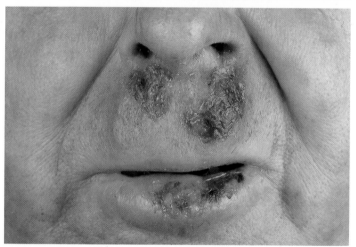

Figure 139. Recurrent herpes simplex in a patient with chronic lymphatic leukemia. Crusty infiltrates of the lips in varying stages of development. The lesions have persisted over a period of months.

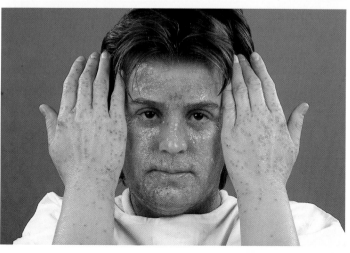

Figure 140. Eczema herpeticum. Rapid exanthematic dissemination of pitted vesicles and erosions over face and dorsum of hands in a woman with atopic dermatitis.

Eczema Herpeticum (Kaposi's Varicelliform Eruption)

1. Densely arranged pitted vesicles rupture after a short time and leave individual widespread erosions.
2. Areas of predilection are face and neck; the entire skin may occasionally be involved.
3. These patients are very ill with a high fever. Serious complications include meningitis, encephalitis, and herpes sepsis; they can be life-threatening. Primary infections are usually more severe than are recurrent manifestations.

Therapy

Treatment of recurrent herpes infections is still unsatisfactory. Therapy is occasionally credited with placebo effects or spontaneous recoveries. At present, it is not possible to eliminate the latent virus from the human organism to prevent recurrent attacks.

Systemic

1. For severe cases of acute herpes infection, eczema herpeticum, and in exceptional cases of recurrent herpes simplex, we recommend Acyclovir (Zovirax intravenously). For less severe cases, Acyclovir may be given orally.
2. Several immunomodulating or immunostimulating substances, such as Isoprinosine (Inosiplex), have been recommended. Their effectiveness in recurrent herpes has not been confirmed, however.
3. A herpes vaccine was available but had to be taken off the market because of its possible oncogenicity. Immunoglobulins to boost the patient's immune system are controversial.

External

1. External application of Acyclovir (R.34) is helpful. Topical commercial preparations of idoxuridine and adenosine arabinoside are much less effective against cutaneous herpes simplex. It is important to apply these substances during the phase of eruption, preferably when premonitory symptoms appear.
2. Pyoderma with crusts is best treated with antibiotic ointments.
3. The patients must be advised not to rub their eyes to avoid autoinoculation. When acute genital herpes is present, condoms must be used for protection.

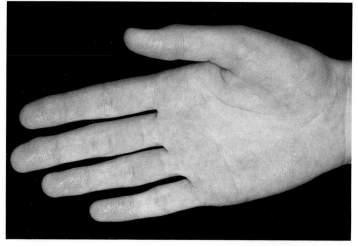

Figure 141. Hyperhidrosis of the palm, most pronounced on the pulps of the fingers.

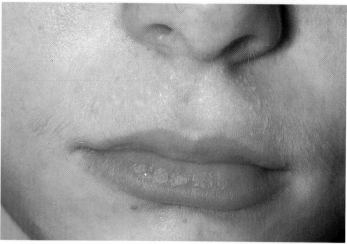

Figure 142. Hyperhidrosis of the lips in a patient with chronic mercury poisoning.

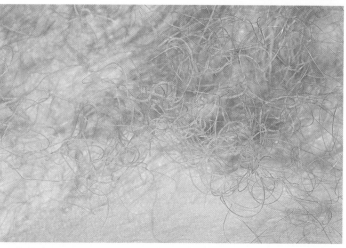

Figure 143. Trichomycosis axillaris. Yellow sheaths on axillary hair in patients with marked hyperhidrosis.

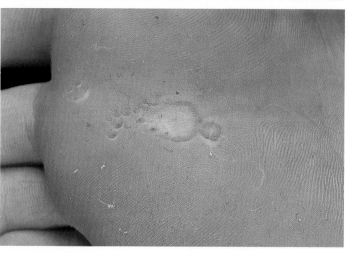

Figure 144. Pitted keratolysis (keratoma plantare sulcatum). "Punched out"–appearing superficial keratin defects on ball of right foot.

Hyperhidrosis and Sequelae

Hyperhidrosis

For practical purposes, we distinguish a generalized or symmetric form from an asymmetric form that is usually due to a neurologic disorder. Generalized sweating is seen in disorders of thermoregulation, infectious diseases such as malaria or tuberculosis; metabolic diseases, such as diabetes mellitus and hyperthyroidism; menopause; malignant tumors (Hodgkin's disease); alcoholism; certain drugs, such as tricyclic and tetracyclic antidepressives, caffeine, theophylline, and cholinergic and sympathomimetic drugs; and chronic mercury intoxication. Emotional factors (fear, stress) can also lead to increased sweating, especially of the palms, soles, axillae, inguinal folds, and face. Some people have a tendency to sweat excessively (genuine hyperhidrosis). Constant excessive sweating can result in unpleasant sequelae such as bromhidrosis (malodorous sweating due to bacterial decomposition) or diseases like miliaria (see p. 99), pityriasis versicolor (see p. 113), trichomycosis axillaris (see below), or pitted keratolysis (see p. 72).

Systemic Therapy

1. Anticholinergic drugs for excessive emotional sweating and mild sedatives may occasionally be indicated. Habit-forming components such as barbiturates must be avoided because this is usually long-term therapy.
2. Extract or tea of sage may occasionally result in improvement.

External Therapy

1. Aluminum chloride in aqueous solution once a day (R.19).
2. For sweaty feet, daily foot baths with potassium permanganate solution (1:10,000) for 10 to 20 minutes can be helpful; this can be combined with oak bark extract (R.8).
3. Surgical sympathectomy is rarely indicated. In hyperhidrosis axillaris, removal of some of the axillary sweat glands is a seldom-used procedure. It must be kept in mind that these are irreversible procedures. Since sweat production diminishes with advancing age, excessive dryness of the skin may result in later years and may be much more distressing.

Trichomycosis Palmellina (Trichomycosis Axillaris)

Marked bacterial invasion of the axillary hair due to hyperhidrosis is characteristic.

Clinical Appearance

There are yellowish-white, firmly attached layers on the axillary hair.

Therapy

1. Treatment of the underlying hyperhidrosis.
2. Frequent use of antiseptic soaps or detergents.
3. Shaving.

Pitted Keratolysis (Keratoma Plantare Sulcatum)

Superficial infection of the skin with corynebacteria is characteristic.

Clinical Appearance

There are multiple superficial roundish defects of the stratum corneum of the soles and the undersurface of the toes associated with hyperhidrosis, maceration, and bromhidrosis. Subjective symptoms are usually minimal. Prolonged mechanical loading (marching), however, can cause considerable pain.

Therapy

The underlying hyperhidrosis should be treated. Severe cases may require a short course of topical antimicrobial therapy (dye solutions, 5% Benzoyl peroxide gel).

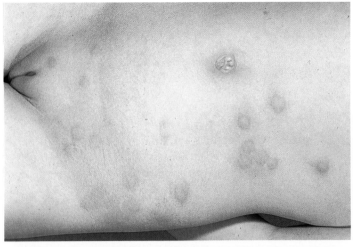

Figure 145. Bedbug bites. Multiple wheals, most pronounced where clothing covers the body tightly.

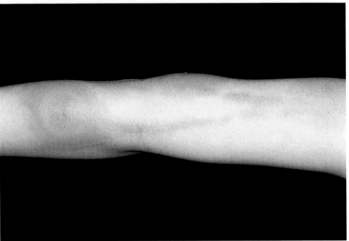

Figure 146. Reaction to an insect bite with lymphangitis. This is usually due to an exaggerated local reaction according to the venom (as in this case) and only rarely due to an infection.

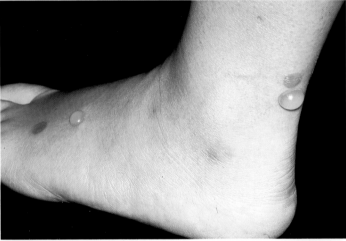

Figure 147. Culicosis bullosa. Bullous reactions to mosquito bites.

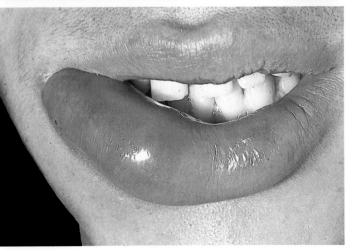

Figure 148. Inflammatory edema of the lips secondary to a bee sting.

Insect Bites

Skin eruptions and occasionally systemic reactions to insect bites occur most frequently during the summer and early autumn. In Europe, mosquito bites and wasp and bee stings predominate; stings and bites from other insects or arthropods, bedbugs, hornets, and spiders are seen less frequently. Flea bites appear to be more common in the United States.

Mosquito Bites

Clinical Appearance

Mosquito bites usually manifest themselves as pruritic wheals or, in some patients, as vesicular reactions, especially on the lower legs.

Therapy

Treatment is not necessary for urticarial reactions. Vesicular eruptions may be treated by evacuation of the blisters. An antibiotic ointment may be applied to prevent infection.

Prophylaxis

1. The patient should try to avoid future mosquito bites: stay away from still waters, do not vacation in mosquito-infested countries, use a mosquito net at night, use no perfumes or cosmetics containing odorous substances, reduce body odor by frequent washing. Mosquitoes are attracted by dark clothing, increased skin temperature, and moisture.
2. Topical repellants afford protection for a few hours.
3. Systemic repellants such as B_1 vitamins (may cause unpleasant body odor) or nicotinic acid have been reported to be effective in some cases.

Wasp and Bee Stings

Clinical Appearance

These stings produce swelling of varying degree around the puncture site. Generalized reactions such as urticaria or even anaphylactic shock are possible. An insect sting into the oral mucosa can lead to a life-threatening edema of the glottis. The clinical appearance following bee or wasp stings varies, and treatment should be administered accordingly.

Therapy

1. *For local reactions*, cooling with moist dressings, dabbing with diluted alcohol (evaporating alcohol has a cooling effect), application of a corticosteroid-containing cream or lotion, and elevation of the affected extremity are helpful. Following a bee sting, the stinger remains in the skin and must be carefully removed without expressing more poison from the poison sac.
2. *For mild systemic reaction* (generalized itching, urticaria), application of a tourniquet proximal to the sting (in extremities), removal of the stinger, and injection of 0.3 ml epinephrine solution (1:1000 in 1 to 2 ml saline [NaCl]) under and around the puncture site are helpful. Antihistamines and corticosteroids can be given intravenously.
3. *For severe reaction* (anaphylactic shock), treatment is determined by the symptomatology: maintain vital functions, positioning, respiratory therapy, and cardiac massage. If necessary, use a slow intravenous injection of diluted epinephrine solution (0.5 ml epinephrine, 1:1000 in 20 ml of 0.9% NaCl solution, given in 0.1-mg boluses), intravenous antihistamines, and corticosteroids.
4. *For stings into the posterior oral cavity* with impending edema of the glottis, the symptoms may be relieved by spraying the oral mucosa with adrenalin aerosol. In severe cases, intubation or tracheotomy may be necessary.

Prophylaxis

1. Later on, it must be determined whether an allergy is present (identification of specific IgE antibodies with RAST). The patient should be warned to avoid stings in the future and should be instructed what to do if stung again.
2. Persons with an allergy should be advised to have an emergency treatment kit at hand at all times, including antihistamines and corticosteroids as water-soluble tablets or solution for intravenous injection, adrenalin-aerosol, adrenalin ampules, tourniquet, and injection kit.
3. If indicated, immunotherapy by an experienced allergist will be necessary.

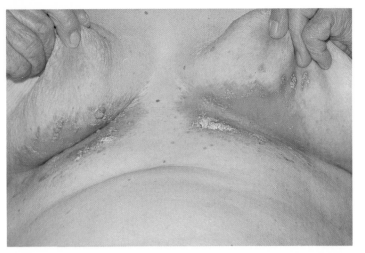

Figure 149. Intertrigo. Sharply delineated symmetric erythema with weeping and crust formation in the submammary area.

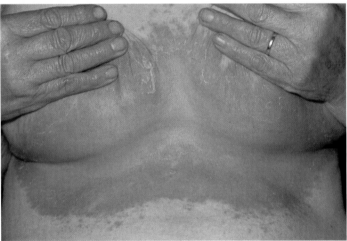

Figure 150. Intertrigo. Widespread erythema and maceration in the submammary area.

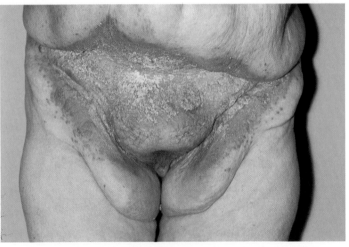

Figure 151. Intertrigo. Extensive involvement in an obese patient.

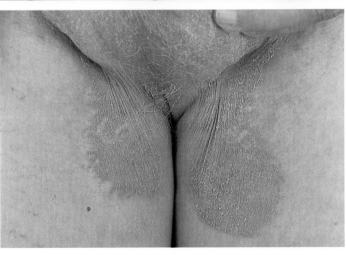

Figure 152. Erythrasma. Sharply delineated, scaling erythema in the inguinal region.

Intertrigo, Erythrasma

Intertrigo

Intertrigo is an inflammation of the skin in those areas where two skin surfaces are in apposition, especially in obese people. Infection with *Candida albicans* (thrush) occurs in all long-standing cases (see p. 109). Hot and humid weather and fever encourage intertrigo.

Clinical Appearance

1. Sharply delineated, widespread, shiny erythema is characteristic. In advanced cases, the erythema can be weeping and itching. It is often covered with scratch marks and crusts.
2. Areas of predilection are the submammary, inguinal, and intergluteal areas.
3. Secondary candidal infection may lead to "satellite lesions," which are disseminated, round, erythematous foci with scaling margins surrounding the main lesion.

Therapy

Symptomatic treatment is rapidly successful in most cases.

For small areas, zinc lotion 2 to 3 times daily is helpful. More pronounced inflammation may require corticosteroid-containing pastes (R.30b) or lotions. For infections with *Candida albicans*, appropriate topical therapy should be used (see p. 109).

Prophylaxis

A bland powder should be used to keep the involved areas dry after intertrigo has healed (R.11). Insertion of linen or gauze strips between the skin folds helps to keep the surfaces separated. The skin should always be dried thoroughly after washing. A fan may be used for the intertriginous areas. Weight reduction is necessary for obese patients.

Erythrasma

This is a common chronic superficial bacterial infection of the skin with *Corynebacterium minutissimum* and affects mainly adults.

Diagnostic criteria are the clinical picture and a coral red fluorescence of the lesions when exposed to UVA light. The disease is harmless and may not require treatment; complications have not been reported.

Clinical Appearance

1. The initially reddish, later brownish, sharply delineated lesions are smooth at first. Later, they show fine plications with mild scaling. Normally there is no pruritus. Itching may indicate eczematization of long-standing lesions, usually in the axillae.
2. Erythrasma is found most often in the inguinal areas and the axillae, as well as in the interdigital spaces of the toes. Typical are symmetric, sharply delineated patches on the thighs close to the scrotum. There are no satellite lesions.

Therapy

Treatment of this harmless disease consists of topical application of creams (R.33a) or solutions (R.14c) containing imidazole derivatives that are also effective against gram-positive bacteria. It may also be treated by topical erythromycin solutions (ATS, Eryderm, Staticin) twice a day for 2 weeks.

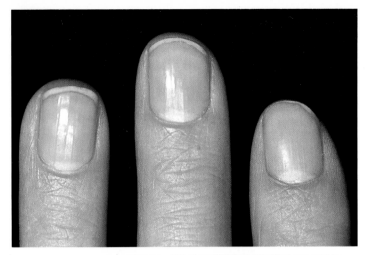

Figure 153. Smoothly polished fingernails from continuous rubbing of the skin to relieve itching.

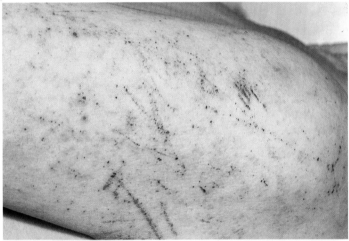

Figure 154. Hemorrhagic scratch lines in a patient with universal pruritus.

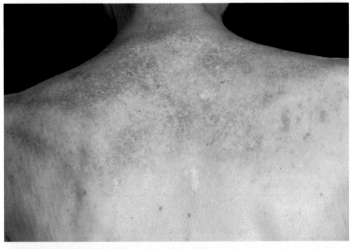

Figure 155. Scratch lines with hyper- and depigmentation secondary to chronic scratching in a patient with generalized pruritus.

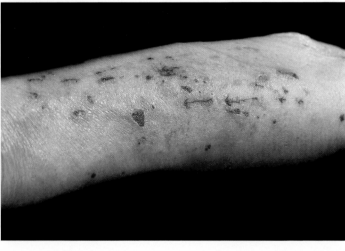

Figure 156. Generalized pruritus in a patient with icterus. Deep scratch marks on the forearm.

Pruritus

Generalized Pruritus

Many skin diseases are accompanied by pruritus. Pruritus can also occur as an independent disorder. Its causes can be harmless ones, such as cold weather, especially in combination with low humidity (central heating), dry skin in older people (see p. 139), and exaggerated body hygiene (excessive bathing and use of alkaline soaps and detergents). On the other hand, many serious internal diseases may be accompanied by generalized pruritus. These include diabetes mellitus, liver and kidney diseases, leukemia, malignant lymphoma, malignant visceral tumors, as well as psychiatric problems (such as delusions of skin parasitosis, and drug abuse). This makes a thorough medical evaluation necessary, unless a trivial cause is evident.

Clinical Appearance

1. Scratch marks, usually from several fingers simultaneously and running parallel to each other, are characteristic. The involved skin is otherwise inconspicuous except for occasional erythema or dryness.
2. Shiny polished fingernails are an obvious indication of habitual scratching.
3. The scratch marks are usually found in areas easily accessible to the hands. Older, less flexible patients often use mechanical aids to scratch other parts of the body.

Therapy

Systemic

A thorough workup to find and treat an underlying disease is necessary.

1. Antihistamines (R.56, R.57), preferably those with a sedative component, are helpful. In these conditions, the advantages of sedation must be weighed against the disadvantages (reduced responsiveness, driving ability, and so on).
2. Sleeplessness may require the addition of a hypnotic (e.g., chloral hydrate).
3. For severe pruritus, antihistamines with a neuroleptic component (Promethazine, Alimemazine) are helpful.
4. For delusions of skin parasitosis, neuroleptic drugs (Haldol, Levomepromazine) can be used. These disorders usually respond to much lower doses than those used for psychiatric diseases.

External

1. There should be regular skin care with lubricants and emollients (R.31b); lubricants may be added to the bath water (R.7).
2. Topical corticosteroid preparations may be used for short periods of time for marked irritation of the skin.

General

1. Excessive washing may have to be reduced.
2. The room climate should be improved (temperature, humidity).
3. Stimulating or hot beverages (coffee, coke, alcohol) should be avoided, especially in the evening.

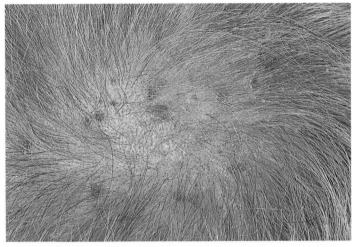

Figure 157. Localized pruritus with round excoriations and impetiginous changes of the scalp. Clinical appearance of "acne necroticans."

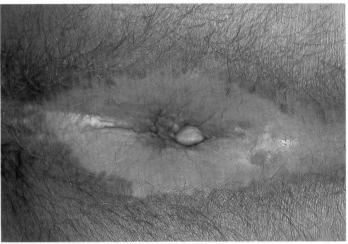

Figure 158. Pruritus ani. Chronic anal eczema with erythema, erosions, hyper- and depigmentation.

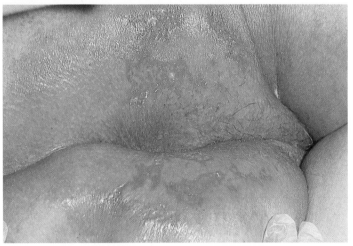

Figure 159. Pruritus ani with extensive erosions secondary to maceration and excoriation.

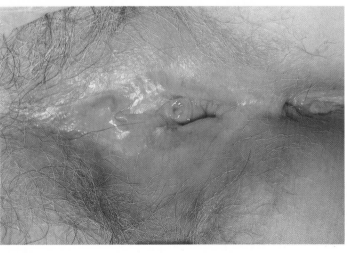

Figure 160. Pruritus vulvae as an essential symptom of genital atrophy in lichen sclerosus.

Localized Pruritus

Several regions of the body are sites of predilection for diseases accompanied by pruritus.

Scalp: seborrheic eczema, psoriasis, pediculosis capitis, acne necroticans.

Periorbital Region: contact eczema caused by cosmetics and airborne allergens.

Nose: hayfever, intestinal parasites in children.

Perianal Region: oxyures (pinworms), dermatomycoses, *Candida* infection, abuse of laxatives, exaggerated anal hygiene, contact allergies to drugs, hemorrhoids, anal fissures, anal or rectal carcinoma, neuroses or psychoses.

Vulvar Region: Candida infection, pubic lice, contact allergies, mental disorders.

Scrotum: Candida infection, dermatomycoses, contact dermatitis.

Legs: chronic venous insufficiency.

In individual cases, those causes mentioned for generalized pruritus can also be responsible for localized pruritus. Dermatoses that cause pruritus can be masked by secondary changes induced by constant scratching, especially in the perianal region, the scrotum, and the vulva, and may not be readily identifiable.

Clinical Appearance

Erythema, scaling, and scratch marks are characteristic, or when scratching is pronounced, even weeping, crusty lesions covered with thick yellowish crusts as a result of bacterial infection. The constant irritation from prolonged scratching due to persistent pruritus may eventually lead to thickening of the skin and even to "elephant skin."

Therapy

As in generalized pruritus, evaluation of possible etiologies followed by causal therapy is the procedure of choice. Recommendations for systemic therapy are the same as those for generalized pruritus (see previous discussion).

External

1. In acute cases, cold moist dressings should be applied for periods of 60 minutes. The dressings should be changed every 20 minutes.
2. Bland lotions or creams or ointments are recommended for chronically dry skin (R.31b, c, d). In exceptional cases, corticosteroids (R.36a, b) may be used for short periods.
3. For pruritus in the anogenital region, sitz baths with tar-containing additions 1 to 2 times a day are helpful.
4. Anesthetic substances (with the exception of pramoxine hydrochloride 1%) should not be used for local therapy; they can cause contact allergies.
5. The skin should be carefully cleansed with warm water and should only be dabbed or fanned dry—no rubbing.

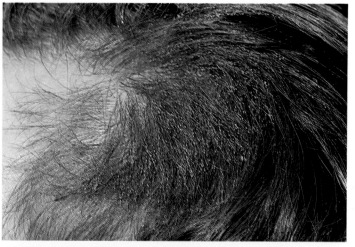

Figure 161. Head lice. Nits attached to the hair in a pearl string–like fashion.

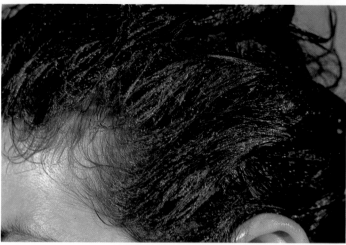

Figure 162. Head lice. Matted hair from massive involvement with nits.

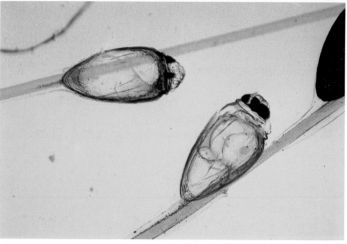

Figure 163. Nits of head lice.

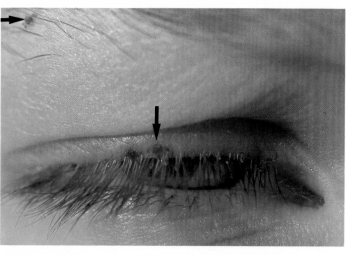

Figure 164. Pubic lice (→). Involvement of upper lid and eyebrow.

Lice

Three types of lice have pathogenetic significance in humans: head lice (pediculus humanus capitis), body lice (pediculus humanus corporis), and pubic lice (pediculus pubis).

Pediculosis Capitis

Head lice are still found fairly frequently today, especially in children. Despite adequate hygienic conditions, epidemic outbreaks occur from time to time, mainly in schools or kindergartens. In these situations, adults can be affected as contact persons; head lice are otherwise rare in adults and are usually found only in neglected patients.

Clinical Appearance

Clinical signs are yellow crusty excoriations with moderate or severe pruritus. Close observation with a loupe reveals rows of nits attached to the hairs. The nits are approximately 1 mm in diameter.

Lice are found less frequently; they are seen in large numbers only in neglected patients. Head lice are found exclusively in the region of the scalp hair, especially behind the ears and in the occipital area. They are approximately 2 to 3 mm long.

Therapy

1. Gamma benzene hexachloride, a pesticide also known as Lindane (Kwell), is the most often used therapy. It is available as a shampoo that is worked into a lather and left on for 4 minutes.
2. The hair is rinsed thoroughly.
3. Retreatment is usually not needed. If live lice are present or eggs are demonstrated at the skin/hair junction at 1 week, a second application may be used.
4. Following this therapy, there is no risk of infection for contact persons. Children can now return to school or kindergarten, even if nits are still visible.
5. Nits are killed by this treatment but continue to adhere to the hairs. The following procedure is recommended for removal of the nits: The hair is thoroughly rinsed with diluted vinegar (ordinary cooking vinegar diluted with water 1:1). The hair should then be wrapped in a moist towel for 30 minutes. The nits can then be removed from the drip-wet hair with a fine-tooth comb, and the hair is then washed with a regular shampoo. This procedure is repeated daily until all nits have been removed.
6. Combs, hair brushes, collars, hats, and bed sheets must be washed or cleaned chemically to avoid reinfection.
7. Contact persons must be examined and treated, if necessary, to avoid epidemic spread of the infestation.

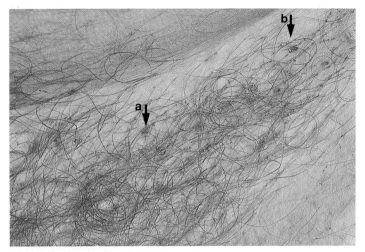

Figure 165. Pediculosis pubis. Pubic lice. Brownish lice (a) that can be recognized clearly only with a magnifying glass and nits glued to the hair (b). Lateral pubic hair.

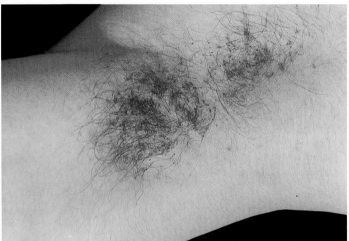

Figure 166. Pubic lice. Involvement of the left axilla.

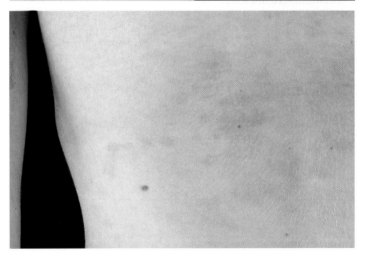

Figure 167. Maculae caeruleae. Pale bluish spots caused by lice bites.

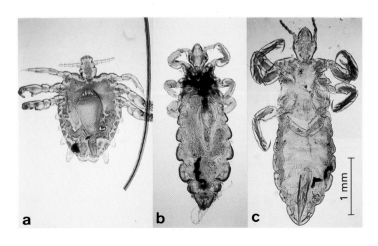

Figure 168. a) Pubic louse, b) head louse, c) body louse. Relative sizes. Magnification 15×.

Pediculosis Corporis

Body lice are close to the body only when they suck blood. One must search for them in the clothing. In today's hygienic conditions, they are found only in neglected persons. The 3- to 5-mm long body louse is significant from an epidemiologic point of view because it transmits rickettsiae and relapsing fever.

Clinical Appearance

1. The bite of the body louse causes marked itching. Deep scratch marks and excoriated papules, at times with pyodermia and hyper- and hypopigmentation, represent the clinical picture of "vagabond's skin" or cutis vagantium.
2. The abnormal changes are found primarily on the trunk, the shoulders, and the gluteal area.

Therapy

1. All infested clothing must be disinfected.
2. Cleansing soap bath and treatment of an existing pyoderma (see p. 123) are helpful.
3. Itching should be treated (see p. 79).
4. Body lice are not found on the body, and therefore, treatment with contact insecticides is unnecessary.

Pediculosis Pubis

Pubic lice are found in all hairy body regions with apocrine glands, especially anal and genital regions, and axillae and occasionally on eyebrows and eyelashes. Pubic lice are transmitted by close bodily contact, mostly during sexual intercourse. They survive outside the human skin for only 1 to 2 days, and therefore indirect transmission is extremely rare.

Clinical Appearance

Maculae caeruleae, pale blue spots of up to fingernail size due to bites, are indicative for pubic lice. They cause moderate to severe itching. The 2-mm long lice and the 1-mm long nits attached to the hairs are easily overlooked on superficial inspection. The lice are normally firmly attached to the hairs and immobile. They can be stimulated to move by careful scratching and are then readily identifiable even without a loupe.

Therapy

1. Lindane lotion or cream is applied to infested areas, except the eyelashes, for 8 to 12 hours, followed by thorough washing. Alternatively, the shampoo can be used as for pediculosis capitis.
2. Eyelash infestations may be treated by applying petrolatum thickly twice a day for 7 to 10 days, with mechanical removal of nits.
3. Examination and, if necessary, treatment of contact persons is important.
4. Clothing and linens must be washed in very hot water or dried on a hot cycle, or both, or dry cleaned.

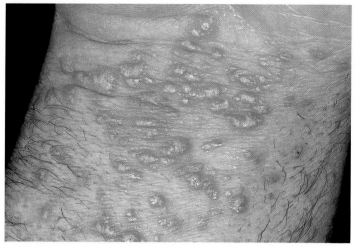

Figure 169. Lichen planus. Polygonal, firm, blue-red papules with somewhat shiny surface (due to reticulated white lines) (Wickham's striae).

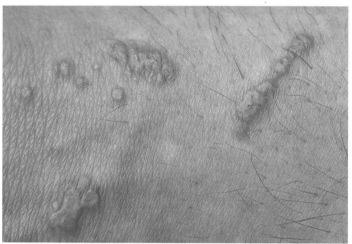

Figure 170. Lichen planus. Köbner-phenomenon. Development of lichen planus papules along a scratch line.

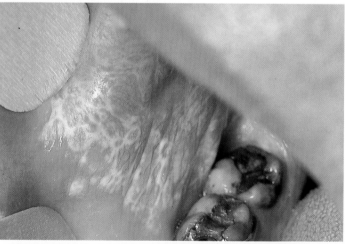

Figure 171. Lichen planus. Pronounced reticulated white coloring of the buccal mucosa.

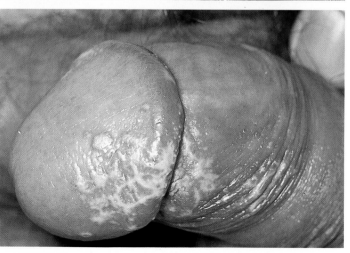

Figure 172. Lichen planus. The same reticular markings on glans penis and prepuce.

Lichen Planus

Lichen planus is a skin disorder that lasts several weeks or months and occasionally several years. It is characterized by widespread eruption of distinctive papules that can coalesce to form larger lesions. The etiology is unknown. In rare cases, the disease can be evoked by drugs (such as gold, pyritinol, or penicillamine) or by organ transplantation (graft versus host reaction). Lichen planus lesions can develop at the site of a skin injury (Koebner's phenomenon).

Clinical Appearance

1. The individual lesion of the disease is a flat, smooth, polygonal papule of dark-red or often bluish-red color (violaceous).
2. The individual papules often coalesce to form larger lesions. Dabbing the papules with oil makes a network of white lines visible (Wickham's striae). Other lesions are ring-shaped (approximately 1 cm), with a raised margin and a depressed, pigmented center. Some lesions are hyperkeratotic.
3. Pruritus is practically always present and is often severe, especially in the initial stage.
4. Areas of predilection are the flexor sides of both wrists, but lichen planus can affect almost any area of the skin. The lesions often appear as individual papules in a rashlike distribution, especially on the trunk.
5. Involvement of the oral mucosa is often observed and confirms the diagnosis. The buccal mucosa shows a network of prominent white lines and occasional erosions. Tongue, gingiva, and lips can also be affected. Sometimes, the oral symptoms are the only manifestations of lichen planus.
6. The genital mucosa is involved less frequently. There, the lesions manifest themselves as a network of white lines that may be raised or appear as ring-shaped lesions.
7. The papules often heal, with a residual pigmentation that can remain on the skin for a long time.

Therapy

Causal treatment is rarely possible. The goal of therapy is to diminish itching and expedite involution of the lesions. Topical treatment takes precedence; systemic therapy should only be considered if local treatment is unsuccessful. Erosive changes of the oral mucosa (precancerous) require treatment and regular follow-up until they are completely healed.

Systemic

1. Treatment is antipruritic; if necessary, antihistamines with a sedative component (R.57) should be used.
2. Etretinate (R.59) is effective, especially for mucosal involvement. Skin changes do not respond quite as well to this medication. Side effects and risks of therapy should be kept in mind.
3. Systemic corticosteroids are effective, but their use is generally not recommended since the lesions promptly recur after the drug is discontinued.

External

1. Topical therapy can be tried with corticosteroid-containing ointments (R.36c).
2. Lesions of the oral mucosa can be treated with corticosteroid-containing lozenges, if available (Betamethasone lozenges), or by dabbing with vitamin A solution (twice a day).

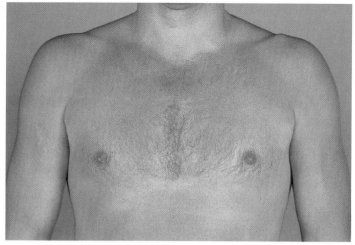

Figure 173. Sunburn, dermatitis solaris.

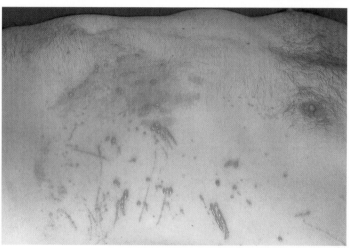

Figure 174. So-called grass dermatitis. Typical vesicular and erythematous streaks, caused by furocoumarins contained in acanthus.

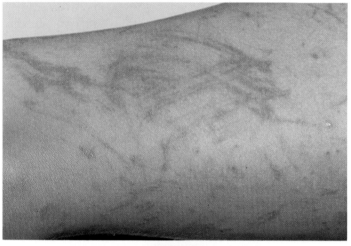

Figure 175. Grass dermatitis. Linear pigmented streaks as sequelae.

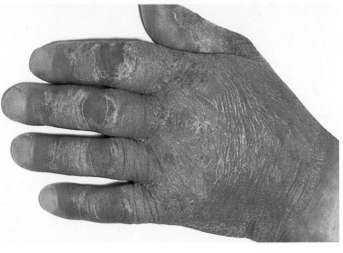

Figure 176. Phototoxic dermatitis. Sharply delineated erythema with scaling.

Light Dermatoses

An overdose of natural or artificial ultraviolet light (UV) causes radiation reaction of the skin of varying degrees, depending on the individual's pigmentation—a sunburn. Sensitivity to light is determined genetically; it is high in persons with blond hair and light skin and very low in Negroes and people of Asian origin. Internal or external use of various substances can also increase sensitivity to light to a point where a dose of UV radiation that would otherwise be tolerated causes an undesirable UV reaction. In addition to these phototoxic reactions, which can be produced in any person, there are certain substances that can cause photoallergic reactions. Furthermore, some skin diseases, such as lupus erythematosus, herpes simplex, porphyria cutanea tarda, and rosacea, can be provoked or aggravated by UV radiation. Finally, there are long-term injuries from prolonged exposure to UV radiation, even if it is below the erythema dose. These injuries include damage to the connective tissue of the skin and induction of actinic keratoses, squamous cell carcinoma, basal cell epithelioma, and melanoma.

Sunburn (Dermatitis Solaris)

Clinical Appearance

1. A mild erythema appears approximately 30 minutes after UV exposure (sunlight, sunlamp). This radiation reaction is followed by a long-lasting pigmentation. Excessive exposure leads to edema and blister formation after several hours, depending on the intensity of the radiation. The maximal reaction is reached after 24 hours and then disappears rapidly. This is followed by desquamation of the skin and later by a long-lasting, occasionally spotty, pigmentation.
2. Only the exposed areas are affected.
3. Pruritus and burning, which can disturb sleep, occur frequently. Severe and extensive sunburn can cause generalized symptoms, such as headache, fever, and even shock.

Therapy

1. Moist, cool dressings are very comforting (R.1).
2. For more severe symptoms, corticosteroid-containing creams or lotions (R.36a, b, c) are useful.
3. In severe cases, systemic administration of aspirin or even corticosteroids may be necessary.
4. Patients who are particularly sensitive to light should use a sunscreen with a high protective factor (R.43) to prevent damage.

Phototoxic Reactions

These are sunburn-like reactions of the skin to a dose of UV radiation (UVA) that would normally be tolerated. The skin reaction is caused by simultaneous external or internal use of a substance that increases sensitivity to light (photosensitizer). These substances include medications, such as tetracyclines; coal tar; or vegetable substances, such as furocoumarins which are contained in plants of the acanthus family or in bergamot oil.

Clinical Appearance

1. Acute dermatitis with erythema, edema, and blister or bulla formation appears a few hours after exposure to UV light.
2. The skin changes are limited strictly to the body regions exposed to the light.

Therapy

Treatment is the same as that for sunburn. In severe cases, systemic corticosteroids (30 to 50 mg prednisolone) are helpful, but doses must be reduced as soon as symptoms have improved.

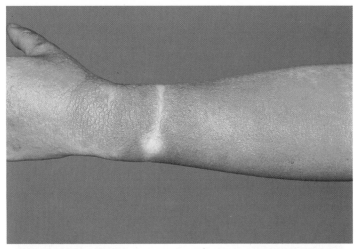

Figure 177. Phototoxic drug reaction. Increased sensitivity to light in a patient being treated with carbutamide. Distinct sparing in the area covered by the wristwatch.

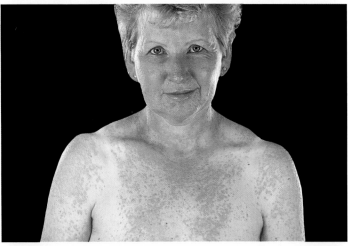

Figure 178. Photoallergic drug reactions from pyrimethamine/sulphadoxine (Fansidar).

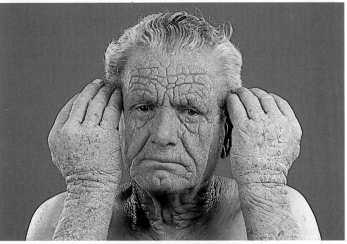

Figure 179. Chronic light reaction, so-called actinic reticuloid. Appearance of chronic eczema with massive thickening of the skin and furrow formation in the light-exposed areas of the body.

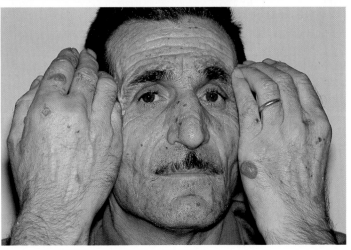

Figure 180. Porphyria cutanea tarda. Blisters and erosions on skin areas exposed to light, especially dorsum of the hand, forehead, and nose.

Photoallergic Reactions

These reactions occur only in sensitized patients upon exposure to light (UVA). Frequent photoallergens are salicylanilides, sulfonamides, and phenothiazine derivatives.

Clinical Appearance

1. The clinical appearance is that of an allergic contact dermatitis (see p. 31). Occasionally, the photoallergic reaction manifests itself as urticaria.
2. The skin changes are most pronounced in the exposed areas but are not as sharply delineated as those in a phototoxic reaction. Occasionally, there can be disseminated papules in the unexposed skin.
3. There is marked pruritus that subsides very slowly.
4. The clinical course is protracted, contrary to that of a phototoxic reaction. It may last several weeks.

Therapy

1. Detection of the photoallergen is of primary importance, if necessary through special tests (photo patch test).
2. A sunscreen that will protect against UVA radiation must be used. One must keep in mind that UVA radiation penetrates window glass.
3. Topical therapy is the same as that for acute contact eczema (see p. 31).
4. Sunlight must be avoided (broad-brimmed hat, long sleeves, gloves).

Persistent Light Reaction, Actinic Reticuloid

If a photoallergy is not recognized early enough, it can result in a persistent light reaction after several years. This means that the symptoms of the disease can be provoked and maintained by light exposure alone, even without an allergen. Actinic reticuloid is the most severe form of a persistent light reaction that is elicited by UV light and also by visible light.

Therapy

Thorough sun protection with opaque sunscreen preparations (Reflecta, RV Paque, zinc oxide cream) and light-tight clothing.

Porphyria Cutanea Tarda

The symptoms of porphyria cutanea tarda could be considered as a special form of phototoxic reaction of the skin. The disease is caused by a disorder of porphyrin metabolism with elevation of the uroporphyrins stored in several organs, including the skin. This disorder is often hereditary. The disease itself is frequently evoked by chronic liver disorders (alcohol, post-hepatic, drug-induced).

Clinical Appearance

After minimal trauma, tense bullae followed by poorly healing erosions and milia develop in areas exposed to light (face and dorsum of the hand). The patient develops dark skin color and hypertrichosis in the face.

Therapy

Internal

1. Phlebotomy therapy with careful monitoring is recommended.
2. Chloroquine, 125 mg two times per week, should be given, with careful monitoring.
3. Alkalinization of the urine and regular monitoring of the urinary pH enhances elimination of the porphyrins.
4. Substances toxic to the liver must be avoided (alcohol, drugs).

External

Sunscreening with pastes or lotions is necessary because maximum absorption of porphyrins takes place in the spectrum of visible light.

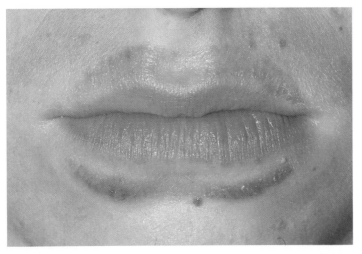

Figure 181. Cheilitis caused by licking. Inflammatory erythema and crusty coatings caused by habitual licking of the perioral area.

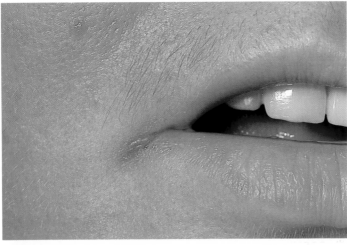

Figure 182. Perlèche.

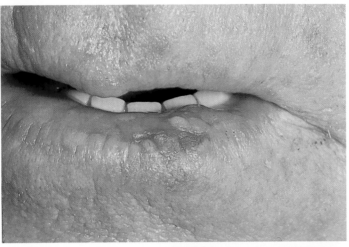

Figure 183. Cheilitis actinica chronica. Erosive crusty lesions and foci of leukoplakia on the lower lip following prolonged exposure to sunlight over many years.

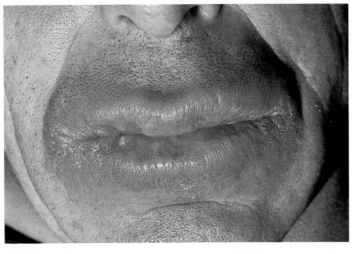

Figure 184. Candida cheilitis. Acute inflammatory erythema and swelling of the lips with erosions and crust formation.

Inflammations of the Lips

Lip-Licking Cheilitis

This is seen frequently in children (often patients with atopic eczema) and is the result of habitual licking of the upper or lower lip, or both, with the tongue or constant moistening with the other lip.

Clinical Appearance

The typical appearance is a sickle-shaped erythema with a raised margin in that area of the lip that can be reached by the other lip or the tongue. Crust formation and secondary infection with bacterial or mycotic organisms *(Candida albicans)* is a frequent finding.

Therapy

Topical treatment is with imidazole derivatives also effective against gram-positive bacteria (R.33a). Treatment has lasting success only if the child's habit can be broken.

Perlèche, Angular Cheilitis

This is a symptom that can have many causes: staphylococcal infections (in children), increased skin creases, hypersalivation, generalized diseases, and poorly fitting dentures. Secondary infection with *Candida albicans* occurs frequently.

Clinical Appearance

Rhagades can be found in the angles of the mouth, at times with eczematization. Pruritus is minimal.

Therapy

Eliminate the causative factors. Topical treatment of *Candida albicans* infection with imidazole derivatives (R.33a) or nystatin (R.33c) for 1 to 2 weeks is recommended.

Cheilitis Actinica Chronica—Chronic Light-Induced Inflammation of the Lips

Chronic damage to the lower lip is often seen in persons who work outdoors. Chronic actinic cheilitis must be regarded as a precancerous lesion.

Clinical Appearance

The red of the lips becomes paler through thickening of the epithelium. The borders between lips and skin become less distinct. The lip is thickened and may be covered with painful erosions or crusts. The lower lip is most often involved, rarely the upper lip. Wind and cold make the condition worse and occasionally produce rhagades.

Therapy

Sunlight should be avoided as much as possible. Topical treatment is with bland ointment bases (R.31a, b); prophylaxis is with sunscreen preparations (R.43).

Thrush-Cheilitis, Candidiasis of the Lips

Extensive thrush infection of the oral mucosa can involve the lips. Clinical appearance consists of swelling and erythema of the lips, occasionally with thickening or rhagades, or both, of the angles of the mouth.

Therapy

The treatment is the same as for other candidal infections (see pp. 109, 111).

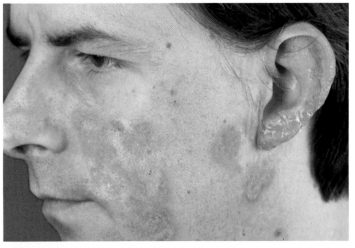

Figure 185. Discoid lupus erythematosus. Extensive infiltrates are slightly atrophic in the center and show markedly enlarged follicle openings. The destruction of the rim of the concha is typical for the disease.

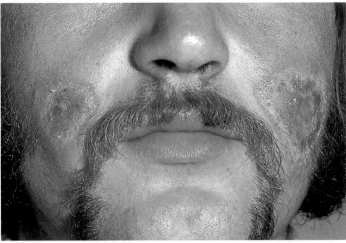

Figure 186. Discoid lupus erythematosus. Discoid lesions with accentuated borders arranged symmetrically.

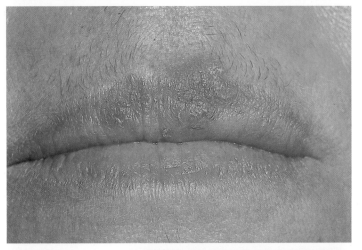

Figure 187. Discoid lupus erythematosus. Persisting infiltrates are spreading to the red of the lips.

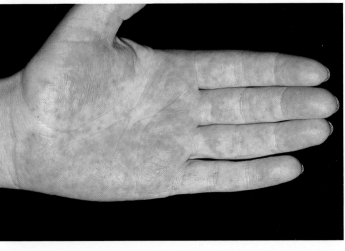

Figure 188. Systemic lupus erythematosus. Bluish-red erythemas of the palm.

Lupus Erythematosus

Two separate forms can be distinguished that occasionally blend into one another:

1. Systemic lupus erythematosus (SLE) is a serious generalized disease involving chiefly internal organs and affecting mainly young women.

2. Discoid lupus erythematosus (DLE) is limited to the skin. Since at first glance it is often impossible to tell which of the two disorders is present, a thorough examination of the entire patient is necessary. DLE is a chronic skin disease that lasts for months or even years. Increased exposure to light as well as prior liver disease foster its development. Antinuclear antibodies, which are characteristic for lupus erythematosus (native DNA, Sm, Ro, and La), are found in the serum of SLE patients.

Systemic Lupus Erythematosus

Clinical Appearance

1. Skin lesions are present in approximately three fourths of all patients. A butterfly-shaped, persistent erythema of the face is typical for the disease. Long-lasting erythematous changes with hemorrhages can often be found in the nail folds. The trunk can exhibit an uncharacteristic macular eruption with maculae of varying sizes. Hemorrhage and ulceration of the oral mucosa can also be found.
2. Symptoms of the generalized disease, such as polyarthritis, polymyositis, nephritis, myocarditis, and pericarditis, as well as psychiatric changes from CNS involvement, often predominate.
3. The patients complain of malaise of varying degree, fatigue, lassitude, and fever attacks.

Therapy

This is a severe and occasionally fatal disease that requires immunosuppressive treatment and often hospitalization of the patient.

Discoid Lupus Erythematosus

Clinical Appearance

1. Erythematous discoid foci with raised borders and a depressed center that exhibits scaling, enlarged follicular openings, and occasionally small keratotic cores are characteristic. The skin is atrophic in these central zones, and a scar remains after the lesion has healed. Less chronic lesions show persistent infiltrates, which look like wheals.
2. Predominantly involved are face and neck, especially the infraorbital region, the nose, and other parts of the face.
3. The infiltrates are painful to touch with the fingernail.

Therapy

1. Symptomatic topical therapy consists of corticosteroid ointments (R.36c), eventually applied under an occlusive foil (see p. 233).
2. External sunscreen therapy is important (R.43).
3. Systemic corticosteroids, immunosuppressive drugs, or cytostatic drugs are normally not necessary in DLE.
4. Systemic hydroxychloroquine (Plaquenil), 200 mg daily, is useful during the sunny season. Patients should be examined regularly by an ophthalmologist to detect retinopathy.

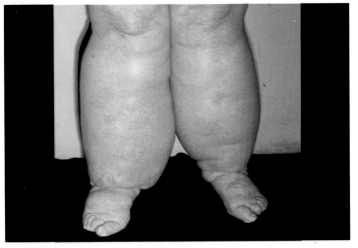

Figure 189. Chronic lymphedema. Elephantiasis. Monstrous persistent swelling following recurrent erysipelas.

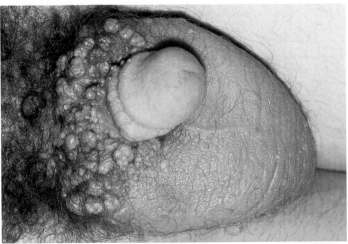

Figure 190. Chronic lymphedema of the scrotum with secondary development of tumor-like dilatation of the lymphatic vessels.

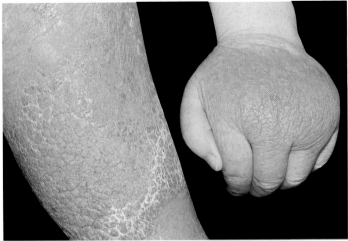

Figure 191. Chronic lymphedema with secondary thickening of the skin, papillomatosis, and induration.

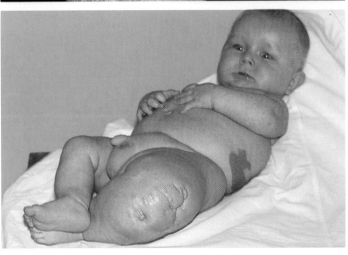

Figure 192. Massive lymphedema in a patient with congenital hematolymphangioma.

Lymphedema

Chronic persistent lymphedema develops where drainage of interstitial fluid is inadequate. The practicing physician usually sees secondary lymphedema. A primary lymphedema on the basis of an inherited hypoplasia of the lymph vessels is very rare. The most frequent cause of secondary lymphedema is chronic, recurrent erysipelas. Other causes are malignant tumors with blockage of the lymph vessels or obstruction of the lymph ducts secondary to operative or x-ray procedures on the lymph nodes, usually in the inguinal or axillary region.

Clinical Appearance

1. Initially there is pitting edema that disappears following elevation of the limb. In longer standing cases, the formation of new connective tissue leads to increasing induration, with warty, sulcated skin and hyperkeratoses. Continued and increasing swelling leads to massive deformity of the affected body regions—"elephantiasis."
2. Lymphedema most frequently involves the legs, the arms, and the genitals.
3. Long-standing edema with increased pressure of the interstitial fluid leads to the formation of small skin-colored tumor-like isolated enlargements of the lymph ducts that resemble condylomata acuminata. They emit lymphatic fluid either spontaneously or when punctured. Widespread, malodorous macerations often develop, with extensive involvement.

Therapy

Possible causes must be evaluated and, if possible, treated.

Systemic

1. Erysipelas, which recurs in short intervals, requires long-term prophylaxis with a depot penicillin for at least several months.
2. All possible portals of entry for a chronic erysipelas must be eliminated (see p. 53).
3. Diuretics are not helpful in the treatment of chronic lymphedema.

External

1. Compression therapy is useful only for lymphedema of the extremities, especially the legs, where it is necessary to prevent the previously mentioned complications.

   This therapy must be carried out with stockings of compression class III or IV. Putting these stockings on is difficult and requires strength. Treatment is effective only when it is done regularly.
2. These measures can be assisted by drainage of fluid either manually or with an apparatus.
3. Surgical reconstructive procedures are only indicated in exceptional cases.

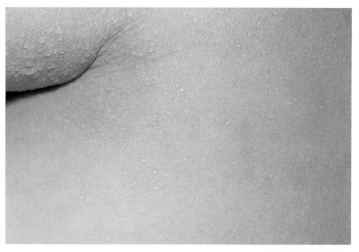

Figure 193. Miliaria cristallina. Disseminated vesicles without inflammatory reaction.

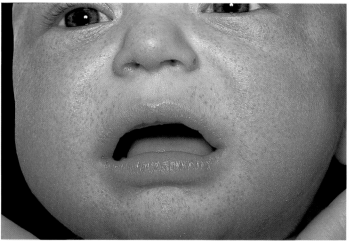

Figure 194. Miliaria rubra. Pinhead-sized, reddened, disseminated papules.

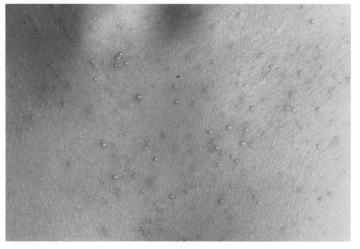

Figure 195. Pustulous miliaria rubra. Disseminated reddened papules and pustules on the upper chest.

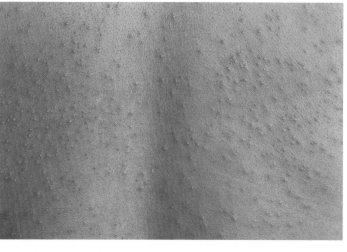

Figure 196. Pustulous miliaria rubra. Dense involvement of the back with papules and pustules.

Miliaria

Miliaria develops as a result of obstruction and rupture of the sweat ducts and pores in combination with marked sweating. Sweat penetrates into the surrounding tissue and causes inflammation. Miliaria is most pronounced during travels into tropical climate zones with high humidity and usually heals spontaneously within a few days after acclimatization. In cooler climates, miliaria is seen mainly after febrile infections. Clothing made of obstructive, usually synthetic, material that does not absorb moisture readily promotes miliaria when the patient sweats. Infants develop miliaria especially when the face is moist with saliva and rests on a rubber mat. Depending on the location of the obstruction, three different forms of miliaria can be distinguished: miliaria cristallina, miliaria rubra, and miliaria profunda.

Clinical Appearance

Miliaria Cristallina

Clear, thin-walled, pinhead-sized vesicles are located under the stratum corneum. There is no inflammatory erythema; the vesicles are found mainly on the trunk. Long-lasting febrile diseases can lead to repeated attacks of miliaria. The vesicles rupture easily and last only for a short time. They are followed by the development of lamellar scales. The patients do not complain of itching.

Miliaria Rubra

The tiny, bright red spots or nodules occasionally have small vesicles or pustules imbedded in them. They usually are widely disseminated. The lesions are found mainly on the trunk and on the flexor sides of elbows and knees, especially under tight clothing. The eruptions cause itching or burning. Itching subsides when the surrounding temperature is lowered.

Miliaria Profunda

This disorder develops as a consequence of recurrent attacks of miliaria rubra and is characterized by pinhead-sized, skin-colored, relatively firm nodules that are localized mainly on the trunk and do not itch.

Therapy

1. The only effective therapeutic measure is the prevention of further sweating. The patient should wear light clothing and avoid hot or stimulating beverages, intensive physical exercise, and tropical climates. Weight reduction is important. For a patient in fully air-conditioned surroundings for at least 8 hours a day, the condition usually heals within a few days.
2. Cooling alcohol dressings and painting with an alcoholic shake mixture (R.20b) will soothe the unpleasant sensations caused by the miliaria rubra eruptions. A bland powder (R.11) can be used on the flexor surfaces of the elbow and knee joints. Topical use of corticosteroid shake mixtures (R.21) is beneficial against inflammation and itching.
3. Excessive use of soap should be avoided.

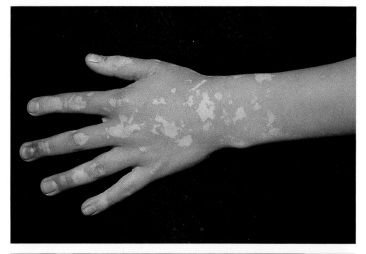

Figure 197. Vitiligo. Symmetrically arranged de-pigmented areas of irregular configuration.

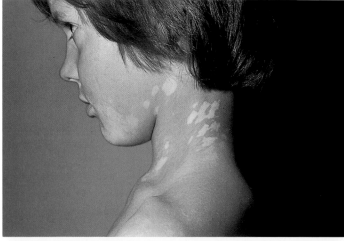

Figure 198. Vitiligo. Similar lesions on the chin and the lateral parts of the neck.

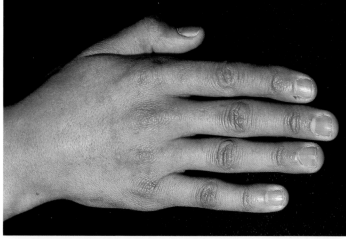

Figure 199. Addison's disease. Diffuse hyperpigmentation, increased over the joints.

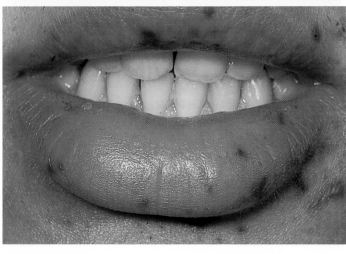

Figure 200. Artificial pigmentation produced by impregnation with silver dust.

Pigmentation Disorders

Vitiligo

Vitiligo is a chronic skin disease that has only cosmetic significance. It is caused by a malfunction of the melanocytes in the epidermis. Familial occurrence is frequent. The disorder can exist in combination with alopecia areata or in patients who have other family members with alopecia areata. The disease persists for years and even decades. In approximately 20 percent of patients, it disappears completely; in another 20 percent, partially. Repigmentation often originates from the follicles.

Clinical Appearance

1. Depigmented, white to rose-colored patches of skin often coalesce to larger areas.
2. The borders are often hyperpigmented.
3. The lesions are usually symmetric and involve mainly the distal ends of fingers and toes, hands and feet. On the trunk, face, and genital regions, the lesions are usually found in the midline.
4. The involved areas are at risk to be sunburned because of the missing pigment protection.

Therapy

Treatment to date is unsatisfactory.

1. In all cases, the use of external sunscreens is indicated on the lesions and on the surrounding skin to protect the depigmented areas from sunburn and to avoid tanning of the healthy skin, which would exaggerate the difference in pigmentation even more.
2. For involvement of the face, application of a water-insoluble makeup is recommended. The cosmetic results of staining the lesions with dihydroxyacetone are often unsatisfactory.
3. Photochemotherapy (PUVA) can be tried in an attempt to achieve repigmentation. This should be done by a dermatologist experienced in the procedure who has the necessary equipment at his or her disposal.

Universal Hyperpigmentation

The disorder has many causes, such as increased excretion of ACTH or melanocyte-stimulating hormone (MSH), as in Addison's disease. This leads to generalized hyperpigmentation with accentuation of the palm lines. Similar changes can be found after prolonged systemic administration of ACTH or other medications such as bleomycin, minocycline, and amiodarone. Melanoma metastases occasionally produce excessive amounts of melanin, which can then be deposited universally. So-called postinflammatory pigmentation, which is a universal pigmentation following inflammatory diseases such as erythroderma, occurs much more frequently. Metallic compounds (mercury, silver) can be deposited in the skin and lead to a brown-grey or blue-grey color. Localized discoloration can be caused by injection or deposition of exogenous particles (injection of metal dust or penetration of dirt in accidents).

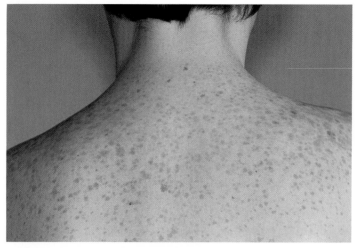

Figure 201. Freckles.

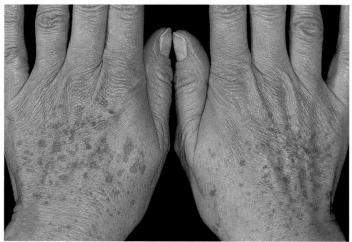

Figure 202. Ephelides of old age. Typical location on the dorsum of the hand.

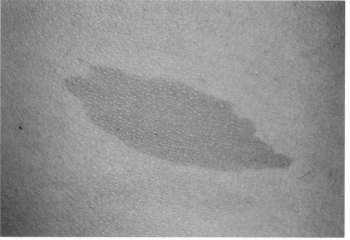

Figure 203. Nevus spilus. So-called "café-au-lait" spot. Sharply delineated light brown spot with homogenous pigmentation.

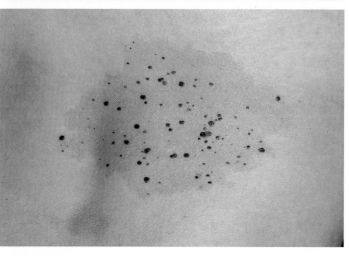

Figure 204. Nevus spilus. Light brown, sharply delineated lesion with multiple interspersed nevus-cell nevi.

Ephelides (Freckles)

Clinical Appearance

1. Disseminated, light brown pigmented spots with a diameter of a few millimeters are characteristic. They occur frequently on constitutionally light skin, which has a tendency to sunburn.
2. Sites of predilection are the face, especially the nasal region, the shoulders, and the back.

Therapy

Treatment is usually not necessary, since this is a harmless normal variant. External application of sunscreen preparations (R.43) may be indicated, as well as hydroquinone-containing creams or lotions (Artra, Eldoquin, Melanex, and so on).

Ephelides of Old Age

These lesions occur in older persons, predominantly on the back of the hand and in the face. They are harmless variants of normal and do not require treatment.

Chloasma

This is a permanent hyperpigmentation of the face caused by estrogen preparations or pregnancy.

Clinical Appearance

1. Spotty or band-shaped symmetric brown pigmentation is characteristic.
2. Chloasma is localized in the face and involves mainly forehead, infraorbital region, and upper lip.
3. The brown discoloration is intensified by UV radiation (sunlight, artificial lamps).

Therapy

1. If the chloasma is caused by estrogens, a nonhormonal method of contraception should be chosen.
2. Excessive exposure to sunlight must be avoided. Application of external sunscreens will protect the skin.
3. Hypopigmentation with hydroquinone-containing agents (Artra, Eldoquin, Melanex, and so on) is helpful.
4. If these measures are unsuccessful, depigmentation should be attempted with a combination of tretinoin, corticosteroids, and hydroquinone (Kligman's prescription). Mercury preparations are no longer recommended. In addition to their toxicity, there is risk of local deposition, which leads to pigmentation as well.

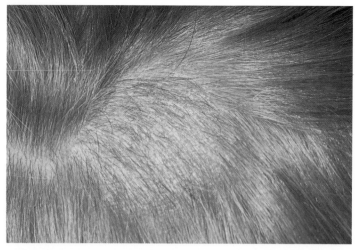

Figure 205. Tinea capitis superficialis. Round "bald" area, with white scales. The stumps of the hairs which have broken off are visible.

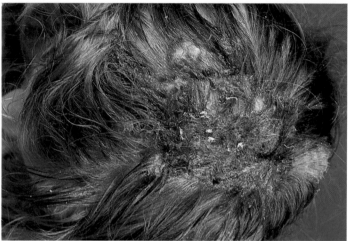

Figure 206. Tinea capitis profunda. Extensive parietal lesions are covered by bloody and purulent crusts. The involved hairs have either fallen out or are stuck together.

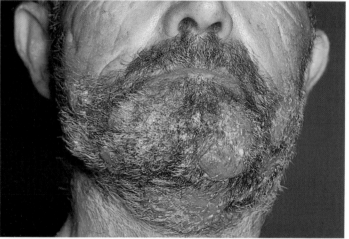

Figure 207. Tinea barbae. Vegetating nodular inflammation with formation of pustules, abscesses, and crusts.

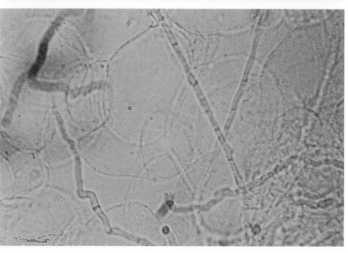

Figure 208. Microscopic demonstration of fungi in the scraping of a scaling lesion after preparation in 10 per cent KOH solution.

Fungal Diseases

Diseases Due to Dermatophytes

Diseases caused by dermatophytes are among the most common infectious diseases of the skin. For practical purposes, it is expedient to classify diseases caused by dermatophytes according to body regions, since the clinical symptoms depend more on the region of the body and the patient's resistance to infection than on the species of the microorganism (frequently *Trichophyton rubrum* and *Trichophyton mentagrophytes*). The diagnosis should be confirmed by microscopic identification of the organism and by culture (on Sabouraud or Kimmig-Agar at 25°C for 3 weeks).

Tinea Capitis

Tinea capitis is classified into tinea capitis superficialis and tinea capitis profunda (Kerion Celsi). Children are affected more frequently than are adults.

Clinical Appearance
1. Tinea capitis superficialis is characterized by round, coin-sized patches without hair that occasionally coalesce into larger areas. There is fine lamellar scaling without inflammatory signs. Stubs of broken hair are visible in the lesion.
2. Tinea capitis profunda presents with marked inflammatory reaction, pustules, crusts, and swelling of the regional lymph nodes. The inflammation originates from the hair follicles, which are infected with fungi.
3. Area of predilection is the scalp; in men the bearded area can also be affected as tinea barbae.
4. The superficial form heals without scars; deep inflammations may result in scarring and alopecia.

Therapy

Systemic
Griseofulvin (R.53) and ketoconazole (Nizoral) (R.54) are equally effective against dermatophytes. The drug should be given for 4 to 6 weeks, depending on the severity of involvement.

Topical
Topical antimycotic therapy alone is not successful against tinea capitis. It can be used in addition to systemic treatment to prevent spreading of infectious material.

Tinea Corporis

Clinical Appearance
1. Sharply delineated, scaling, erythematous lesions with wavy accentuated borders and formation of pustules, especially along the margins, are characteristic. The lesions enlarge slowly in a peripheral direction. They may be aggravated by sunlight.
2. Lesions can develop anywhere on the body. Pets (cats, dogs, guinea pigs) can transmit the infection to exposed skin areas (face, arms), especially in children. Furthermore, other lesions can be found in the gluteal and inguinal areas (tinea cruris).
3. The infection causes moderate to severe itching.

Therapy

Internal
Griseofulvin (R.53) and ketoconazole (Nizoral) (R.54) are very effective, but external therapy alone is adequate for tinea corporis and is preferable.

Topical
1. Local antibiotics in a base appropriate for skin type, location, and degree of inflammation can be used in a solution (R.14b, c) or a lotion or cream (R.33a, b) for at least 2 to 3 weeks.
2. Aqueous dye solutions (R.14a) have an antimycotic effect but stain the underwear and should not be used on an outpatient basis.
3. Corticosteroids are not recommended. They have an anti-inflammatory effect but encourage dissemination of the fungi on the skin.

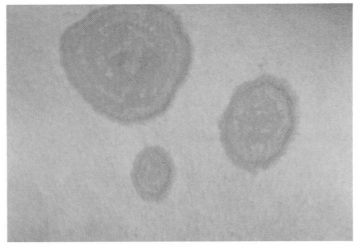

Figure 209. Tinea corporis. Sharply delineated erythemas have a zonal arrangement with scaling and pustule formation along the margins.

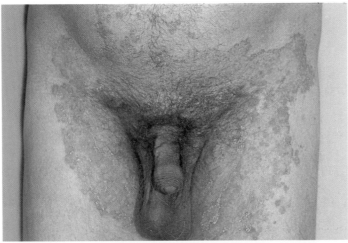

Figure 210. Tinea cruris. Scaly, partly infiltrated erythema with polycyclic borders that enlarges peripherally. The accentuated margin is typical for the disease.

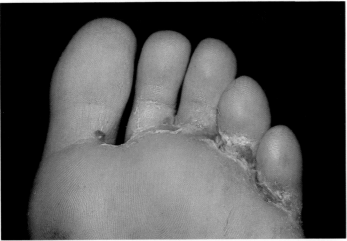

Figure 211. Tinea pedis. Maceration with erosions and scaling originating from the interdigital spaces.

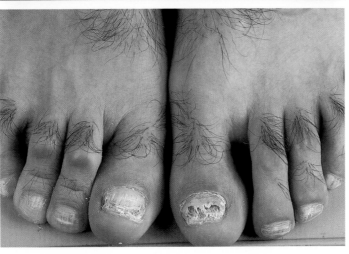

Figure 212. Onychomycosis, tinea unguium. Thickening, whitish-yellow discoloration and partial destruction of the toenails.

Tinea Pedis

Clinical Appearance

1. Scaling, erythema, maceration, and rhagades are found between the toes.
2. The skin changes are found most frequently in the fourth interdigital space with occasional spreading to the dorsum of the toes and the soles of the feet. The toenails are often involved.
3. The patient usually complains of itching in the involved area. Prolonged wearing of athletic shoes or rubber boots can produce the effect of a moist chamber, especially in patients with hyperhidrosis, and lead to acute exacerbation with severe inflammation and dyshidrosis ("athlete's foot") (see p. 29). Acute erysipelas (see p. 53) can also originate from tinea pedis.

Therapy

1. Use appropriate foot wear. Avoid rubber boots and tight shoes; wear sandals and cotton socks instead. The interdigital spaces must be kept dry (bland powder).
2. Foot baths with antimycotic additives (potassium permanganate [R.4]) are helpful. Dry thoroughly after bathing; use a fan.
3. Antimycotic powders (R.13) or solutions (R.14) can be used; insert gauze strips between the toes.
4. Systemic antimycotic therapy is usually not indicated in tinea pedis. Secondary bacterial infection or erysipelas requires appropriate antibiotic treatment.
5. To avoid reinfection, contaminated socks must be washed in very hot water. Disinfection of contaminated footwear is also necessary.

Tinea Unguium, Onychomycosis

Constant work in a moist environment damages the nail plate and encourages fungal infection. The patient often suffers from poor peripheral circulation (smoking, acrocyanosis) or arterial occlusive disease. Usually, onychomycosis is a harmless disorder, and therapy is not always necessary.

Clinical Appearance

1. Whitish-yellow discoloration of the nail plate starts at the free end of the nail and advances slowly toward the nail bed. This is followed by thickening and loosening of the nail plate from the nail bed. Finally, the nail becomes brittle.
2. The toenails are affected more frequently than are the fingernails.

Therapy

Mycoses of the nail are very resistant to therapy and recur frequently. It is advisable to inform the patient of these problems before treatment is started. If blood supply is poor, attempts should be made to improve it, otherwise antimycotic therapy will not be effective. Before systemic medication is started, the organisms must be identified microscopically and by culture since onychomycosis can be caused not only by dermatophytes but also by yeasts and saprophyte fungi.

Systemic

1. Griseofulvin is helpful in the treatment of dermatophytes (R.53) (6 months for fingernails; 10 months for toenails). Onychomycoses recur frequently, despite adequate treatment.
2. In long-term therapy, ketoconazole (Nizoral) can have undesirable effects on the liver and is, therefore, no longer recommended for onychomycosis.

Topical

1. The thickened nail is softened with 15 per cent urea-containing ointment, followed by treatment with an antimycotic (R.25). Treatment must be continued until a healthy nail has grown. This therapy is successful only occasionally, even with regular and prolonged application.
2. Extraction of the nail is usually not successful because the fungal infection recurs readily. Damage to the nail matrix during extraction can result in growth of a defective nail, which is even more susceptible to fungal infection.

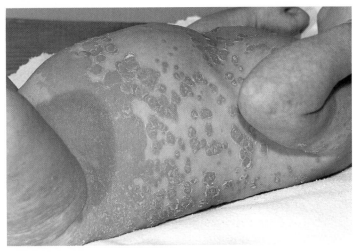

Figure 213. Candidiasis (thrush) originating from diaper rash. Sharply delineated scaly erythema tapers off into multiple satellite foci. Distinct squamous margin.

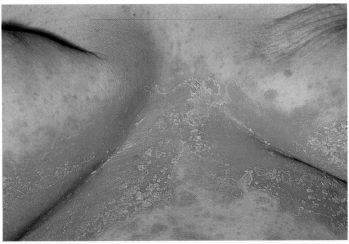

Figure 214. Candidiasis (thrush). Scaly erythemas with a solid red color and marginal scaling. Satellite foci in the periphery.

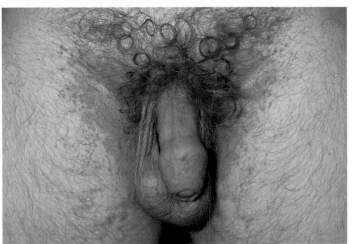

Figure 215. Candidiasis (thrush). Largely symmetric erythema, tapering off into individual foci, located in the inguinal area, and extending to the scrotum.

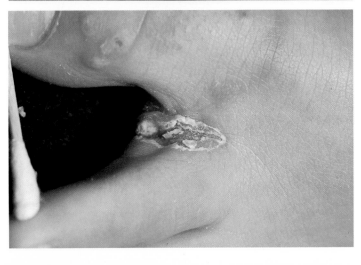

Figure 216. Candidiasis (thrush). Typical development in the interdigital space. Rhagade covered with scales.

Skin Diseases Caused by Yeasts (Candidiasis)

Candida albicans is the primary pathogenic yeastlike fungus. These infections involve the intertriginous areas, the nailbed, and occasionally the mucous membranes. Candidiasis can occur as a primary disease but is more often secondary to treatment with broad-spectrum antibiotics, corticosteroids, or cytostatic agents. It also occurs in diabetes mellitus and serious illnesses that impair the immune system (malignant lymphoma, collagen diseases, pemphigus). These patients may develop life-threatening sepsis following fungal infection of the skin or mucous membranes. Ordinarily, candidal infections are found only in newborns or infants and elderly and debilitated patients. Chronic candidal infections are seen mainly in patients with congenital or acquired defects of cellular immunity.

Candidal Infection of the Skin

Clinical Appearance

1. Bright red, smooth, macerated lesions in the intertriginous areas are characteristic. Small papules with scaling scalloped borders (satellite lesions, typical for candidal infection) are found in the periphery.
2. Cutaneous candidiasis occurs predominantly in the intertriginous areas, such as the perianal region, the inguinal area, the submammary area, the axillae, and the interdigital spaces. In a patient with an impaired immune system, candidal infection can exceed these locations and involve the entire skin.
3. The patients often complain of burning and pruritus.

Therapy

Elimination of the causative factors is of prime importance, especially the increased moisture of the skin found in patients with marked sweating (obesity, fever), incontinence, and diabetes mellitus.

Systemic

1. For extensive involvement and in patients with increased risk (leukemia, cytostatic treatment), systemic use of ketoconazole (R.54), one tablet daily for 1 to 2 weeks, is recommended.
2. Confirmed intestinal candidiasis is treated with nystatin or amphotericin B orally. (These two substances are not absorbed and are locally effective.)

Topical

1. The intertriginous areas should be kept dry with powder or zinc lotion and the insertion of gauze strips between the toes.
2. Sitz baths with antimicrobial additives such as potassium permanganate are helpful, followed by drying with a fan.
3. A paste containing nystatin (R.29) is very effective. Ointments are not an advisable vehicle for intertriginous areas.
4. Dye solutions (R.14a) are acceptable for the perianal region and the vulva and are very effective there.
5. In infants, occlusive diapers should be avoided in favor of linen diapers.
6. Reduction of dietary intake of sugar is recommended as an additional measure.

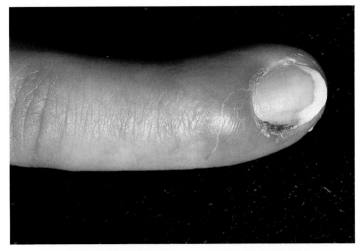

Figure 217. Candidiasis with paronychia. Clinically this acute periungual inflammation cannot be distinguished from a bacterial infection.

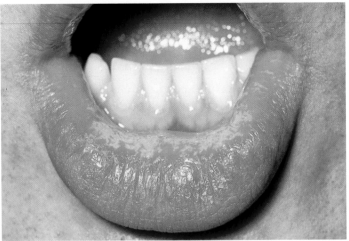

Figure 218. Candidiasis, oral thrush. The reticulated white plaques are located on the periphery and can be scraped off.

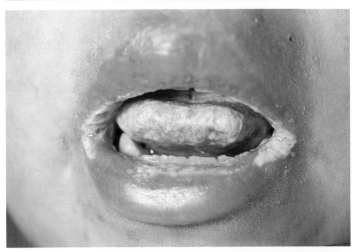

Figure 219. Chronic muco-cutaneous candidiasis in a patient with cellular immunodeficiency. Thick white coating of the tongue and in the corners of the mouth (thrush-perlèche) and the red of the lips.

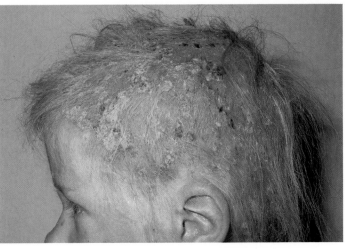

Figure 220. Chronic mucocutaneous candidiasis in a patient with cellular immunodeficiency. Extensive inflammatory infiltration of the scalp, which is covered with crusts.

Candidiasis of the Mucosa, Candidiasis of the Genital Area

Clinical Appearance

1. Creamy white, adherent plaques of approximately pinhead to small coin size are characteristic. They can coalesce to widespread membranous plaques.
2. The mucous membranes of the mouth and the tongue may be affected. Similar changes can occur as candidal vulvovaginitis on the female genitals and as candidal balanitis in the male. In patients with an impaired immune system, the *Candida* infection can spread from the oral mucosa to the pharynx and esophagus.
3. In candidal balanitis, round or circinate bright red, smooth lesions on the glans penis and on the prepuce of the penis are characteristic.
4. When perianal or perivulvar candidiasis is present, intestinal or vaginal infection must be suspected and appropriate diagnostic studies and, if necessary, appropriate treatment instituted.

Therapy

Mucosal Candidiasis

1. Treatment with a suspension of an antimycotic drug (nystatin, amphotericin B, miconazole) is helpful.
2. In severe cases that are resistant to the previous therapy, ketoconazole (Nizoral), 1 to 2 tablets for 5 to 10 days may be helpful.
3. Continued prophylaxis with ketoconazole during immunosuppressive therapy in patients with AIDs may be indicated.

Genital Candidiasis

1. Most antimycotic drugs have a similar effect on the treatment of vaginal infection. They are applied as vaginal suppositories or vaginal creams.
2. External application of a cream containing nystatin (R.33c) or imidazole compounds (R.33a) can be helpful.
3. Sitz baths with potassium permanganate solution soothe the severe pruritus.
4. Simultaneous intestinal candidiasis should be treated.
5. In genital candidiasis, treatment of the sexual partner is necessary to avoid "ping-pong infection."

Candidal Paronychia

Clinical Appearance

1. The skin surrounding the fingernail will show marked discoloration and edematous swelling. Pressure on the tissue produces thick purulent material. The cuticle is absent. Chronic infection causes impaired growth of the nail and occasionally yellow-green discoloration. (This may indicate secondary infection with *Pseudomonas aeruginosa*.)
2. In persons who work in a moist medium (dishwashers, cleaning personnel, hairdressers), the fingernails are more frequently involved than are the toenails.
3. Chronic paronychia often leads to impaired growth of the nail with transverse ridges on the nail plate.
4. The patient should always be evaluated for diabetes mellitus.

Therapy

1. Elimination of the predisposing factors is of prime importance. Rubber or vinyl gloves worn over cotton gloves will avoid a moist chamber effect on persons who work in a wet medium. This work must be avoided completely during the acute phase of the disease. The cuticle must not be manipulated.
2. Antimycotic drugs in solutions or tinctures (R.14c) transport the effective agent to the infected lesion.
3. Hand baths for short periods of time only can be helpful for patients with marked purulent secretion.
4. Consistent application of these measures usually results in marked improvement, but it may take 2 to 3 months.
5. Short-term treatment with ketoconazole is indicated only for massive infections resistant to other treatment. The infectious organism must be identified before treatment is started.

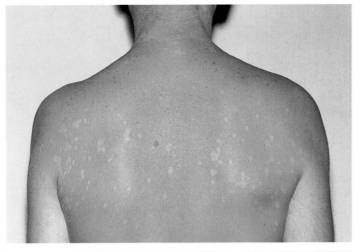

Figure 221. Pityriasis versicolor. Oval-shaped, hypopigmented, minimally scaling lesions are located along the relaxed skin tension lines.

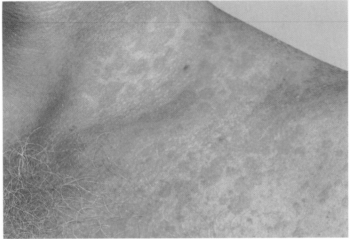

Figure 222. Pityriasis versicolor. On a light skin the round, confluent, brownish foci can be distinguished well.

Figure 223. Pityriasis versicolor. Clinical appearance in detail.

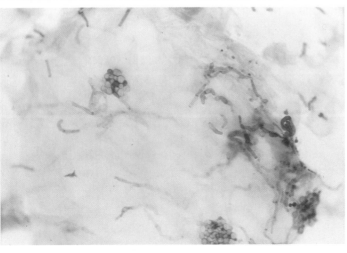

Figure 224. Identification of the causative organism *(Pityrosporon orbiculare)* with azur-stained cellophane tape preparation. Microscopic examination shows a typical mixture of round yeast cells and hyphae.

Pityriasis Versicolor

Pityriasis versicolor is a noninflammatory, noncontagious fungal disease caused by the bimorphic yeast *Pityrosporon orbiculare* (ovale). This fungus occurs naturally as a saprophyte on the skin. It produces a substance that interferes with melanin synthesis (azelaic acid). Therefore, the affected areas are of a lighter color, in contrast to the surrounding tanned skin. On a nontanned skin, these areas appear light brown.

Pityriasis versicolor occurs more frequently during the summer and in hot, humid climates. The disease is also found as an accompanying phenomenon during systemic corticosteroid therapy, in patients with immunodeficiency syndromes, or during immunosuppressive therapy. Poor body hygiene does not seem to be a factor. Patients more than 40 years of age are rarely affected.

Clinical Appearance

1. Flat, round or oval-shaped lesions that can occasionally coalesce to palmsize lesions are characteristic. Scraping with a wooden spatula produces branlike scales. The color of these lesions may range from white to red or brown.
2. The lesions are found mainly on the shoulders, chest, back, and occasionally the upper arms and thighs.
3. The disorder is mainly a cosmetic problem with occasional mild pruritus. The scales can be removed by Scotch tape, and the causative fungi can be identified by staining with blue ink, gram stain, or methylene blue solution. Direct microscopic examination of scales from scrapings shows short hyphae and clusters of budding yeasts.

Therapy

With all therapeutic measures, one must keep in mind that the disease recurs readily and is only a cosmetic problem.
1. The most important therapeutic measure is elimination of the underlying hyperhidrosis.
2. Pyrithion zinc cream (R.10) is applied to the whole body, including the scalp (a fungus reservoir), and removed by thorough showering. This is repeated every other day for 14 days.
3. Selenium IV sulfide (Selsun) is just as effective but may be toxic when applied to large areas (significant resorption).
4. Topical broad-spectrum antimycotics (R.33a) are also effective but must be applied 1 to 2 times daily for at least 3 to 4 weeks, which can be expensive.
5. Systemic ketoconazole is effective but is not indicated for this harmless disorder.
6. It is important to inform the patient that it will take 2 to 3 months or renewed suntanning before the pigmented lesions regain the same color as the surrounding skin.

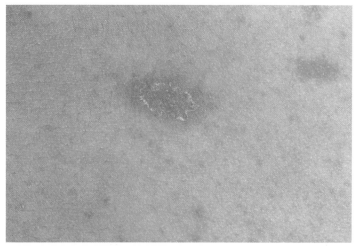

Figure 225. Pityriasis rosea. Fairly large initial lesion with scaly margin (so-called herald patch).

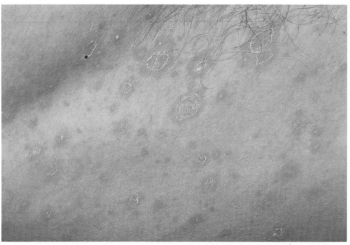

Figure 226. Pityriasis rosea. Exanthematic dissemination of round and oval-shaped erythemas of various sizes with characteristic collarette scale.

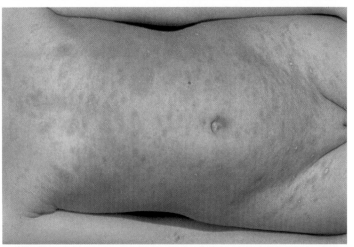

Figure 227. Pityriasis rosea. Maximal development of the disease with herald patch, and lesions oriented in the direction of the relaxed skin tension lines. Typically, only the trunk and the proximal parts of the extremities are involved.

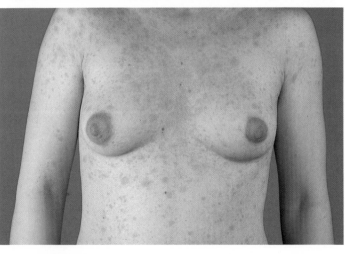

Figure 228. Pityriasis rosea. Exanthema involving mainly the trunk. The usual scaly border is absent.

Pityriasis Rosea

The cause of this common, nonrecurrent disease is unknown. A virus etiology is suspected because the disease usually occurs during the spring and because of other epidemiologic hints. Pityriasis rosea has a characteristic appearance and a typical location (see later) that is important for the diagnosis. It develops slowly to the full-blown picture over a period of 5 to 10 days and lasts approximately 3 to 6 weeks. Young adults, adolescents, and children are affected most frequently. Pityriasis rosea— like eruptions are known to occur after treatment with certain drugs, such as Captopril, Clonidine, and gold.

Clinical Appearance

1. The first symptom usually is a 2 to 5 cm, round or oval, reddened, scaling lesion with an accentuated border, the so-called "herald patch," which is generally found on the trunk.
2. Several days to 3 weeks later, symmetric eruptions of similar but smaller pale red to pinkish-brown lesions with silvery scales appear.
3. The lesions are located on the lateral and anterior parts of the trunk, especially on the chest. With more extensive involvement, they can also be found on the proximal parts of the extremities. The patches are often oblong, with the long axis running parallel to the relaxed tension lines of the skin. A collarette is usually found between the center and the margin of the individual focus. Pale red patches without collarette appear simultaneously.
4. The face and the distal parts of the extremities are rarely involved.
5. Pruritus is minimal and is present only occasionally.
6. A secondary eczema is often found in the affected region. The skin of these areas can be irritated easily, e.g., by cortisone ointments. This can retard healing.

Therapy

1. The disease usually disappears spontaneously after 3 to 6 weeks, even without treatment. Therapy is not required in most patients, but mild topical therapy with a zinc lotion (R.20a, c) may be useful.
2. Topical corticosteroids are not beneficial, except a shake mixture for severe inflammatory lesions.
3. Pruritus may be managed with oral antihistamines (R.56, R.57).
4. UVB therapy appears to have a direct beneficial effect on both the pruritus and the extent of the eruption.
5. Other measures such as corticosteroid ointments, frequent washing with soap, and wool clothing should be avoided because they irritate the eruptions and retard healing.

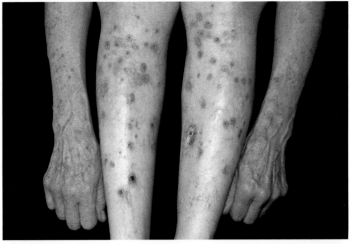

Figure 229. Prurigo. Nodules with circumferential inflammatory reaction on the extensor aspects of the extremities, which have been scratched open due to intense itching.

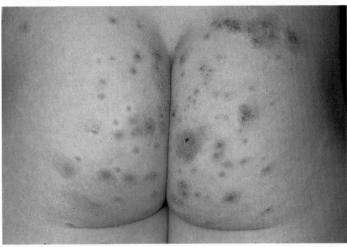

Figure 230. Prurigo. Acutely inflamed, mostly excoriated nodules in the gluteal region.

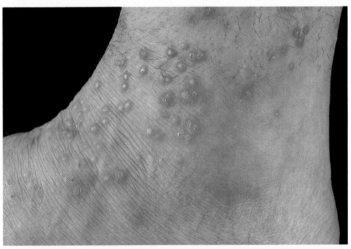

Figure 231. Prurigo. Firm, markedly pigmented and intensely itching nodules of long duration.

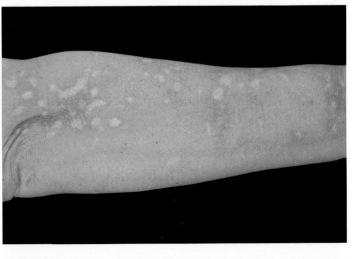

Figure 232. Prurigo. Residual scarring. Round, depigmented lesions with hyperpigmented margins.

Prurigo

This term defines a special mode in which the skin reacts and is characterized by severely itching papular eruptions. There is no recognizable local cause. In some cases the development of skin changes is followed by marked pruritus; in other cases, the lesions are caused by constant scratching. Evaluation must include a thorough workup for possible systemic diseases: diabetes mellitus, impaired kidney function, liver diseases, hematologic disorders, helminthic infection of the intestines, and drug abuse.

A skin disease caused by parasites (scabies, lice) must be excluded. Prurigo can be a late manifestation of atopic dermatitis in adolescents and adults (see p. 47). In many patients, the cause of prurigo cannot be found, despite a thorough evaluation. The disease can run a short and acute course, especially in children, but can also have a prolonged and chronic course over many years.

Clinical Appearance

1. The primary lesion in prurigo is a firm seropapule (a wheal-like reaction topped by a small vesicle). The vesicle is usually removed by scratching and is visible only in the beginning. More often, one sees lentil-size, centrally excoriated, papules; later, one may occasionally find deep, punched-out ulcerations.
2. Prurigo occurs mainly on the extensor sides of the extremities, less frequently on the trunk, and on the face. The palms, the soles of the feet, and the mucous membranes are not involved.
3. The lesions heal, with often long-lasting hyper- or depigmentation. Deep excoriations result in permanent scars. Prurigo papules on the lower legs can be especially tenacious.
4. The excoriations are restricted to the prurigo papules, which is typical for prurigo; linear excoriations are rare. Characteristically, patients report that the massive spotty pruritus is reduced significantly immediately after lesions are scratched open.

Therapy

1. Clarification of the etiology is of prime importance. In those cases in which the etiology can be found, the underlying disease must be treated. If a neuropsychiatric problem (delusions of skin parasitosis) is suspected, evaluation and treatment by a psychiatrist are indicated.
2. Antihistamines are useful for the treatment of pruritus, especially those with a sedative component (R.57). For severe cases, neuroleptics in low doses may be indicated (e.g., haloperidol [Haldol] 5 drops 3 times per day).
3. A topical anesthetic in a vehicle appropriate for the condition of the skin may be helpful (lotions for acutely irritated skin, pastes and especially ointments for long-standing lesions without irritation of the surrounding skin), occasionally with the addition of a tar preparation (e.g., ictasol [Ichthyol] 5%, liquor carbonis, detergens 5%, or ichthammol [Tumenol] 5%).
4. Corticosteroid ointments (R.36a, b) should be used only for severe inflammatory, eczematous reactions.
5. Intralesional injections of corticosteroids (R.44) can be helpful for persistent, circumscribed lesions.

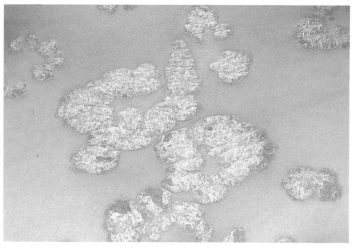

Figure 233. Psoriasis vulgaris. Sharply demarcated, scaling, reddened, individual round plaques.

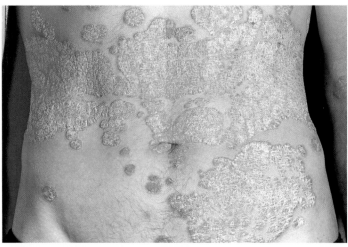

Figure 234. Psoriasis vulgaris. Individual lesions coalesce to widespread figurate lesions.

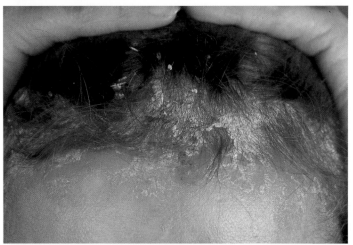

Figure 235. Psoriasis vulgaris. The lesion involves the scalp with typical ribbon-like extension to the forehead.

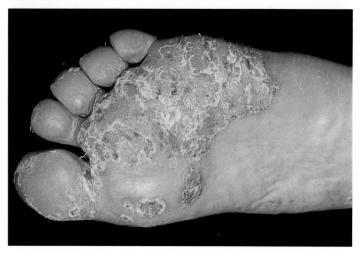

Figure 236. Psoriasis vulgaris. Involvement of the sole of the foot with development of pustules, which can be seen frequently in this location.

Psoriasis

Psoriasis is one of the most frequent skin diseases in the United States, with an estimated prevalence of 1 to 2 per cent. The tendency to develop psoriasis is inherited; the cause of the disease is unknown. The disease can manifest itself at any age, most often in young adults, less frequently in children and elderly patients. The course of the disease varies considerably in individual patients. It usually runs an extremely chronic course with phases of remission and exacerbation. Certain factors may provoke psoriasis. These factors vary with individual patients. They include external factors such as irritation of the skin by pressure, injuries, and sunburn. Psoriasis can also develop in pre-existing skin diseases like drug eruptions, allergic contact dermatitis, or other eczematous diseases. This characteristic tendency of the skin of psoriatic patients to react to external stimuli with the development of psoriatic lesions is known as isomorphic response or Koebner's phenomenon. Endogenous factors may also provoke development of psoriasis. These include chronic alcohol abuse; mental stress; certain drugs, especially beta blockers and lithium; chronic infectious diseases, acute and recurring tonsillitis, and obesity. Patients with psoriasis are usually in good health unless they develop an acute exacerbation (for instance, pustular psoriasis, psoriatic erythroderma) or psoriatic arthritis. The cosmetic disfiguration, however, often reduces the quality of life significantly and may lead some patients to become alcoholics or even to commit suicide.

Clinical Appearance
Psoriasis Vulgaris

1. Infiltrated erythematous patches of varying size (mostly lentil- to palm-sized areas) sharply delineated from the surrounding skin with a round or oval or polycyclic border are characteristic. The lesions are covered with thick, imbricated and adherent whitish scales that can be removed with the fingernail as a small chip (like chips from a wax candle). Pinpoint bleeding occurs when a scale is picked off. This is typical for psoriasis and is known as Auspitz sign.
2. Psoriasis has a predilection for the elbows, knees, scalp, and sacral areas.
3. The fingernails are frequently involved and show pitting, with the appearance of oil droplets when subungual keratoses are present, onycholysis, and heaped-up subungual debris. In advanced cases, the nail plate may be lifted off its bed, the nail becomes brittle and crumbles, and the paronychium is involved.
4. Subjective symptoms are usually absent. Occasionally, the lesions become irritated and itch, especially on the scalp and in the intertriginous areas.

Pustular Psoriasis

The spectrum of this type of psoriasis extends from chronic pustular involvement of palms and soles (psoriasis pustulosa, type Königsbeck-Barber) to generalized development of pustules on the entire skin with a severe, occasionally life-threatening, course (psoriasis pustulosa, type von Zumbusch). Psoriasis pustulosa can develop from psoriasis vulgaris, or it can develop suddenly without prior psoriasis.

Psoriatic Arthritis

This is a chronic, destructive arthritis in patients with psoriasis and involves mainly the interphalangeal joints, the spine, and the large joints. Rheumatoid factors are negative. Skin lesions, or at least changes in the nails, are usually present. Prolonged involvement can lead to marked joint deformities.

Erythrodermic Psoriasis

Psoriasis can develop secondarily into erythroderma, in which the entire skin is erythematous and shows massive scaling. A prolonged course of this disease can lead to significant fluid and protein losses. The patients may be severely ill. The disease can be caused by irritating topical treatment, especially excessive UV radiation.

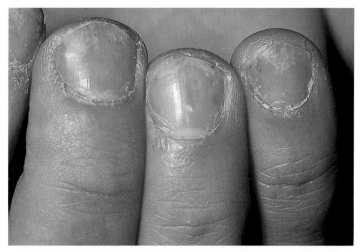

Figure 237. Psoriasis vulgaris. Involvement of the nails with dimple-like pits and oil stain–like discolorations that emanate from the free end of the nail. The discolorations can cover a large part of the nail.

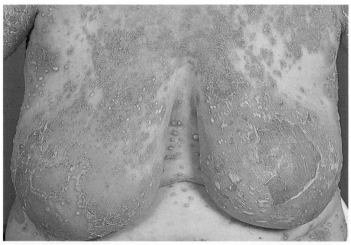

Figure 238. Pustular psoriasis. Acute disease with pustules on a widespread circinate erythema. There is extensive desquamation of the upper layers of the epidermis on the left breast.

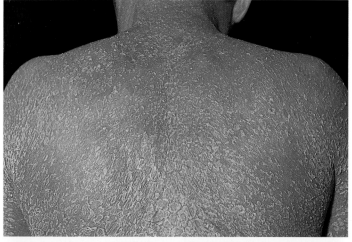

Figure 239. Psoriatic erythroderma. Universal involvement of the skin with erythema, scaling, and thickening of the skin.

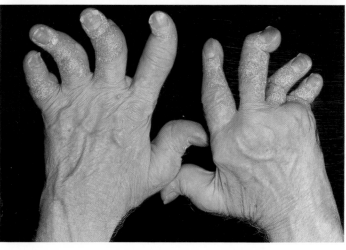

Figure 240. Psoriatic arthritis. Marked deformity of the fingers with significant limitation of motion. Skin and nails show typical psoriatic changes.

Therapy At the present time, there is no cure for psoriasis. Therapeutic measures can only produce a remission of symptoms. At best, the psoriasis can be converted from an active to a latent state, with diminished scaling and itching, and the cosmetic appearance can improve. The unpredictable course of psoriasis produces phases in which intensive therapy is necessary. At other times, the patient is practically free of symptoms and no treatment is required. The patient may need psychologic guidance during the long course of the disease. It is especially important that he or she learns to mistrust so-called "miracle cures."

Systemic Systemic therapy must be limited to patients with severe disease whose symptoms cannot be kept under control with other measures.

1. Retinoids, especially Etretinate (R.59) have a very good antipsoriatic effect, especially against psoriasis pustulosa, psoriatic erythroderma, and psoriatic arthritis.
2. Corticosteroids can be used systemically and topically with good results. When treatment is discontinued, there is usually an exacerbation of symptoms (rebound phenomenon), occasionally to a severe form (psoriasis pustulosa). It is for this reason that systemic corticosteroids should be used only in exceptional cases.
3. Certain cytostatic drugs, especially methotrexate, have a good antipsoriatic effect. Since the introduction of retinoids, however, they are indicated only in those cases in which all other measures have failed.

Topical 1. It is very important to remove the thick layer of scales with salicylic Vaseline (3 to 5%) and with baths to which soft soap has been added.
2. Anthralin (1/64 to 2%) (R.35) appears to be the best topical antipsoriatic drug. High concentrations lead to skin irritation and dermatitis; the optimal dose must be found by starting with a low dose and carefully increasing the concentration. The substance has the added disadvantage that its oxydation products cause lasting stains on underwear and sanitary equipment. Attempts have been made to modify Anthralin therapy (Short Contact Anthralin Therapy [SCAT]) in order to reduce these undesirable side effects. Anthralin therapy requires great therapeutic experience, especially when dealing with widespread psoriasis. These patients should always be referred to a dermatologist who has adequate knowledge of this therapy.
3. Tar products (R.37d, e) have a distinct antiproliferative effect. The disadvantages are the unpleasant odor and the staining of skin and clothing; bituminous coal tar causes increased photosensitivity.
4. *Corticosteroids.* In general, corticosteroids cannot be recommended as the primary topical therapy of psoriasis. It is true that they produce a rapid remission of the psoriatic lesions, but the lesions recur as soon as treatment is discontinued. The chronic character of psoriasis requires long-term therapy, which may lead to undesirable corticosteroid side effects. With topical treatment of extensive lesions, systemic effects can occur from resorption of the drug through the skin. Local treatment with corticosteroids is indicated for certain sites, however. Corticosteroid-containing tinctures (R.18) are helpful for psoriasis of the scalp and the auditory canal. Corticosteroid creams (R.36a, b; R.37b, d) are useful on the face and in intertriginous areas for short periods of time.
5. *UV therapy.* The effectiveness of ultraviolet light on psoriatic skin lesions has been known for a long time. UV therapy is carried out as selective ultraviolet therapy (SUP) with long wave UVB light or as photochemotherapy, which is a combination of a photosensitizing drug such as 8-methoxy-psoralen (methoxsalen) and UVA light (PUVA). Because of the possible risks involved with photochemotherapy, the method should only be used by an experienced dermatologist who has the necessary equipment at his or her disposal. UV therapy requires relatively little time. Topical treatment is not necessary with its use, except for lubrication of the skin and removal of scales before UV therapy is started. Treatment must be continued for a long time; the risks regarding carcinogenesis following artificial long-term UV radiation of the skin are still under discussion.
6. Psoriasis in the stage of eruption should be treated with relatively mild measures (no Anthralin, no photochemotherapy, no fatty ointments).
7. Psoriasis of the scalp is treated like a seborrheic dermatitis (see p. 37). Additionally, an occlusive foil and a shower cap may be used at night to enhance penetration of the active medication.

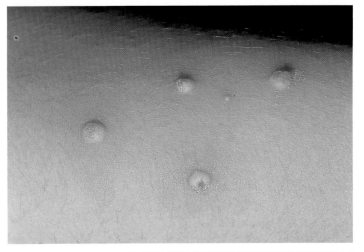

Figure 241. Follicular pustules. Purulent inflammation of the hair follicle. Pustules with surrounding erythema.

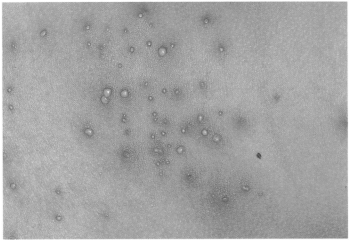

Figure 242. Follicular pustules. Extensive dissemination of pustules surrounded by inflammatory reaction.

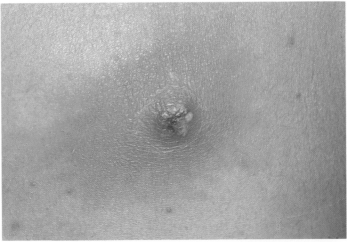

Figure 243. Furuncle. Acute inflammatory tumor with central purulent core. The lesion is surrounded by individual pustules.

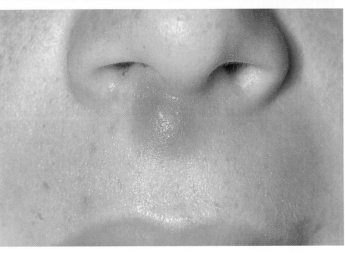

Figure 244. Furuncle at the entrance to the nose.

Pyodermas

Folliculitis, Follicular Pustules

Follicular pustules are infections usually caused by *Staphylococcus aureus.* Single or multiple follicular pustules (infections of the pilosebaceous apparatus) can be caused by a variety of factors: local or systemic impairment of the immune system, increased or changed bacterial flora of the follicles, systemic diseases (e.g., diabetes mellitus), or fatty skin due to constant contact with oil or prolonged treatment with fatty ointments. Follicular pustules can develop into furuncles.

Clinical Appearance
1. Follicular pustules are often pierced by a hair and surrounded by a small erythematous zone.
2. These pustules appear only in those areas of the skin that have hair follicles. Therefore, they do not develop on the palms and the soles. Pustules occur most frequently on the chest, back, and extremities.

Therapy
Before treatment is started, it is important to evaluate the patient for systemic or local causes, underlying diseases, or occupational exposure to oil, and so on.

1. The pustules may be evacuated and dabbed with a disinfecting solution (R.17); 1% Rivanol lotion may also be helpful.
2. The bacterial flora of the skin can be reduced by frequent washing with detergents (R.5).

Furuncle and Furunculosis

A furuncle is a deep-seated infectious folliculitis and perifolliculitis with a purulent core. Furuncles develop in patients with transient or permanent local or systemic impairment of the immune system. They often occur as single lesions. Other patients may develop recurrent furuncles over a prolonged period of time (recurrent furuncles, furunculosis). This disease affects mainly young men who are otherwise healthy. The patients must be evaluated for a variety of factors: alcoholism, drug abuse, diabetes mellitus, leukemia and other malignant diseases, AIDS, and chronic diseases of the liver.

Clinical Appearance
1. The slightly raised inflammatory erythema with a central core undergoes central necrosis and pus formation within a few days. The core usually ruptures and drains, but the furuncle can also be resorbed and regress without rupturing.
2. Trunk and extremities are affected most frequently; the face is involved occasionally.
3. Lymphangitis and enlargement of the regional lymph nodes occur. In rare cases, sepsis can complicate the course of the disease.

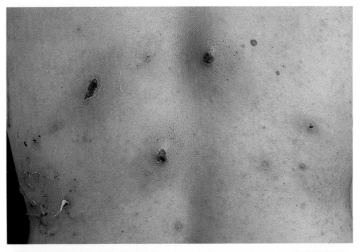

Figure 245. Furunculosis. Multiple furuncles in a patient with diabetes mellitus.

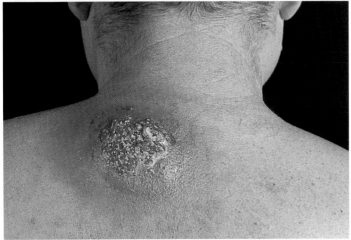

Figure 246. Carbuncle on the neck. Severe involvement with extensive, acutely inflamed swelling and multiple small purulent foci.

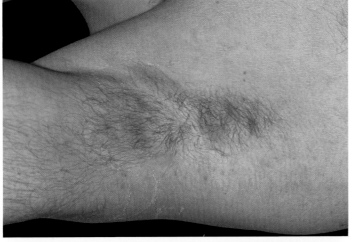

Figure 247. Abscesses of the sweat glands. Painful nodular inflammation in the right axilla.

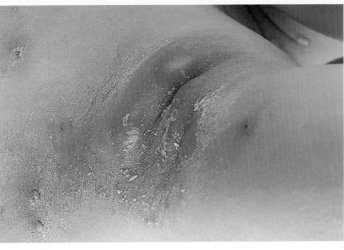

Figure 248. Abscesses of the sweat glands. Painful, nodular and abscess-forming inflammation in the left axilla surrounded by individual pustules.

Therapy	Local therapy is sufficient in most cases. In furuncles of the nose and upper lip, the infection may spread through the vena angularis with resultant sinus thrombosis or meningitis. They require special therapeutic measures.
General	Patients with systemic symptoms, with impaired immune systems, and especially with furuncles of the face should be on bedrest. For furuncles of the nose and upper lip, there should be no speaking and no chewing.
Systemic	1. Furuncles of the face must be treated with systemic antibiotics. Furuncles in other sites require parenteral antibiotics only when generalized symptoms or impairment of the immune system are present, then, penicillinase-resistant antibiotics like oxacillin or dicloxacillin are preferable. 2. For recurrent furuncles, treatment with an immunostimulating substance or an auto-vaccine therapy can be tried. 3. Substitution of immunoglobulins is indicated only in patients with antibody deficiency.
Topical	1. Ichthyol ointment (R.39b), covered with a dressing, can be helpful. 2. Cold application (ice cubes) enhances resorption in the early stages. 3. Local heat application (infrared light) induces hyperemia and expedites suppuration. 4. When abscess formation has occurred, it should be drained with a stab incision. 5. Application of topical antibiotics to the anterior nares is used in recurrent lesions to eradicate carrier states.

Carbuncle

The special anatomic situation at the back of the neck favors these painful inflammatory processes, which are aggregates of furuncles.

Therapy	In addition to the measures outlined for furuncles (see previous discussion), generous incision under general anesthesia is usually necessary to drain the pus.

Sweat Gland Abscesses

These abscesses are found mainly in the apocrine glands of the axillary, inguinal, perianal, and perigenital regions. Multiple, recurrent sweat gland abscesses (so-called hidradenitis suppurativa) are usually a symptom of acne conglobata and frequently occur in patients who show other symptoms of acne conglobata (see p. 5).

Clinical Appearance	1. Nodular swellings with and without pus formation are seen. In severe cases, inflammatory erythema occurs later, with formation of fistulae and irregular, cordlike scarring. 2. The areas of predilection are the axillae, inguinal, perianal, and perigenital areas. 3. In advanced cases, the abscesses can be painful.
Therapy	Treatment is difficult in many cases. The abscesses tend to recur over a prolonged period of time. Minor surgical procedures (incision of abscesses, excision of small nodules) are often performed but should be avoided if at all possible. They usually do not prevent a recurrence and often cause keloid formation, which makes the condition worse. If conservative therapy is not successful (see later), major plastic surgery with excision of the entire involved area, followed by plastic closure of the defect (e.g., latissimus dorsi plasty), is the procedure of choice. These are technically difficult operations and are indicated only for severe scar formation.
Systemic	1. Isotretinoin (R.60) is the most effective treatment for advanced cases. 2. Treatment with parenteral antibiotics (tetracyclines in descending doses) as recommended for acne (see p. 5) is less effective. 3. Treatment with immunostimulating substances (see earlier) has been tried with little or no success.
Topical	Topical therapy contributes little because the changes are located deep in the dermis. Washing with disinfectant soaps reduces the bacterial flora of the skin.

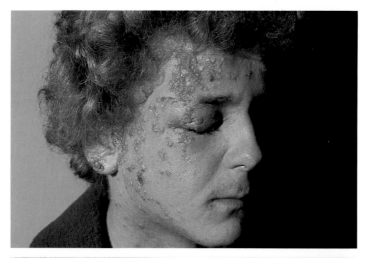

Figure 249. Impetigo contagiosa. Yellow crusts and pustules in a planar or circinoid distribution. The skin is otherwise unchanged.

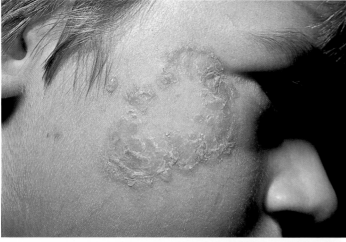

Figure 250. Impetigo contagiosa. Annular lesion with layered, yellow, crusty coating.

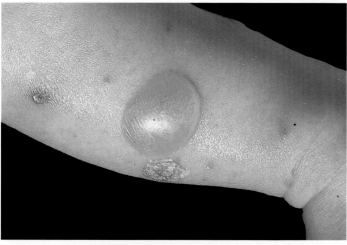

Figure 251. Impetigo contagiosa. Bullous form of the disease, often seen in children.

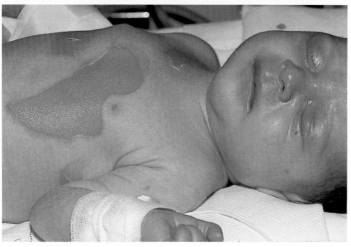

Figure 252. Staphylococcal scalded skin syndrome (Ritter's disease). Bullous infantile impetigo in its maximal form. Bullae or remnants of bullae with extensive desquamation of the upper epidermis.

Impetigo Contagiosa

Impetigo contagiosa is the most frequent bacterial skin disease in children. The diagnosis is usually easy, and therapy is rapidly successful in most cases. This superficial skin disease is caused by streptococci or, less frequently, by staphylococci. The infection is transmitted by direct skin contact and develops rapidly. Several children in one family are often involved (contact infection). The children should be kept out of school or day care for several days to avoid spreading the disease. Impetigo occurs more frequently in children who live in poor socioeconomic conditions, but this does not necessarily imply that the disease is generally due to lack of cleanliness. Children with atopic eczema have a tendency to develop impetigo. Impetigo occurs more frequently in hot and moist climates. Complications of impetigo-like glomerulonephritis or sepsis are rare today. Impetigo should not be confused with secondary bacterial infection (impetiginization) of pre-existing skin diseases, such as scabies, eczema, or insect bites.

Clinical Appearance

1. Golden yellow to dark yellow layered crusts form round, centrifugally enlarging lesions. These lesions often have a distinct margin, or the crust is present on the margin only, so that the lesions are irregular, with curved borders and an erythematous base.
2. Occasionally, vesicles and erosions predominate instead of crusts.
3. Areas of predilection are the face and occasionally the intertriginous areas (axillae, inguinal region), but the disease can affect any part of the body.
4. Moderate pruritus is present. There are no systemic symptoms.

Therapy

Topical therapy is usually promptly effective and normally sufficient.

1. Antibiotic ointment such as polysporin is applied after washing with Betadine or Hibiclens.
2. A disinfectant full bath (R.4) also helps to loosen the crusts.
3. Systemic antibiotic therapy is only necessary for widespread vesicular impetigo or when septic complications are present.

Staphylococcal Scalded Skin Syndrome

This severe form of vesicular staphylococcal impetigo can develop very rapidly in small children. It usually occurs as a secondary disease after a bacterial infection such as otitis media. The extensive vesicle formation is caused by staphylococci of group 2, phage type 3A, 3B, 3C, 55, and 71.

Clinical Appearance

1. The disease is characterized by large bullae, ruptured bullae, and erythema.
2. The entire skin can be involved. The bullae are found predominantly in areas exposed to mechanical forces, pressure areas and areas where the skin is frequently moved (eyelids, and so on).
3. This is a severe generalized disease with high fever and fatigue. The patients often have difficulty drinking. Immediate hospitalization is necessary.

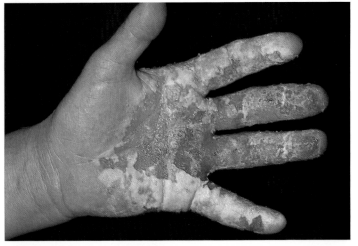

Figure 253. Acute radiation dermatitis. Acute erosive-ulcerative inflammatory radiation reaction after radiation accident.

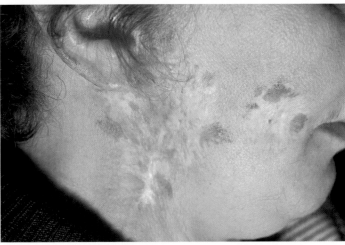

Figure 254. Radiation dermatitis. Figurated scar corresponding to the irradiated field. Adjacent to it are remnants of the irradiated nevus flammeus.

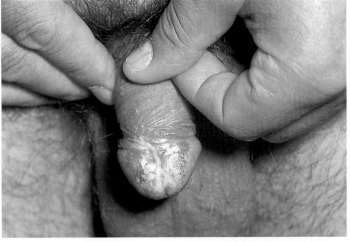

Figure 255. Radiation dermatitis. Firm, patchy fibrous scarring with telangiectasias.

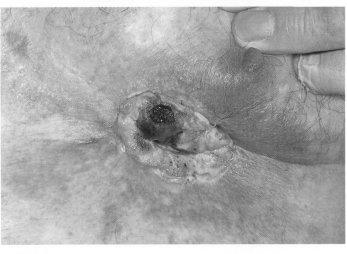

Figure 256. Squamous cell carcinoma secondary to radiation dermatitis.

Radiation Damage to the Skin

Irradiation of the skin with ionizing radiation (roentgen rays, grenz rays, beta rays, and gamma rays are used for medical purposes) causes dose-dependent damage to the skin. Acute radiation dermatitis consists of an inflammatory reaction due to the direct cell injury. Chronic radiation damage to the skin occurs after multiple exposures to low-level radiation as a summation effect. These changes can be due to local radiation to the skin or to deep irradiation of internal organs.

Radiation damage to the skin is seen less frequently today, because radiation treatment of the skin, especially for benign and inflammatory disorders, is not used very often, and better methods for deep irradiation of internal organs (rotational irradiation, fast electrons) have been developed.

Acute Radiation Dermatitis

Clinical Appearance

This acute reaction of the skin to ionizing radiation is classified into three stages according to the degree of severity. The mildest form (first degree acute radiation reaction) consists of erythema, appearing after 1 week, followed by hyperpigmentation, which lasts for a prolonged period of time. Higher doses produce a more intensive inflammatory reaction, with edema, blistering, and long-lasting erosions (second degree acute radiation reaction), which is always followed by permanent scarring. The most severe form of acute radiation injury to the skin is characterized by complete tissue destruction and deep necroses. After demarcation, an ulcer develops that is very resistant to treatment (third degree acute radiation reaction). This type of radiation reaction is always the result of an overdose of radiation and is never a desired therapeutic effect.

Therapy

An undesired acute radiation reaction can be treated with topical corticosteroids to combat inflammation. Systemically, pain medications with anti-inflammatory action, such as aspirin or other nonsteroidal anti-inflammatory drugs, are given.

Chronic Radiation Dermatitis

Clinical Appearance

This stage develops following second and third degree acute radiation dermatitis and also as a result of a high total radiation dose that was given in fractionated low-level individual doses. After a latent period of 2 to 10 years, the skin becomes thin and vulnerable, with telangiectasias, spotty hyper- and depigmentation, and thickened connective tissue (radiation fibrosis). Deep, poorly healing ulcers develop in the center of these areas even after mild trauma (radiation ulcer). In addition, one sees keratotic changes (radiation keratosis). Radiation ulcers and radiation keratoses can eventually lead to radiation carcinoma, the most severe complication of radiation injury. Suspected lesions should always be evaluated by biopsy.

Therapy

1. Topical therapy of roentgen dermatitis consists of frequent lubrication of the skin with a mild ointment (R.31b, c) and protection from mechanical injury to prevent the development of ulcers.
2. Long-standing radiation ulcers that fail to heal, especially those with malignant changes, must be treated surgically by excision. These procedures are technically difficult and not without risk, especially when the radiation fibrosis extends to the bone.
3. Topical corticosteroids should be avoided in cases in which the skin is already thin and friable.

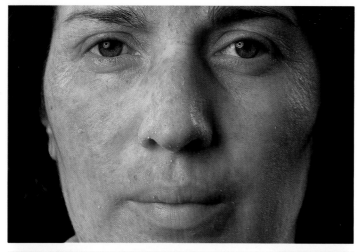

Figure 257. Rosacea. Disseminated papular form involving the face and the eyelids.

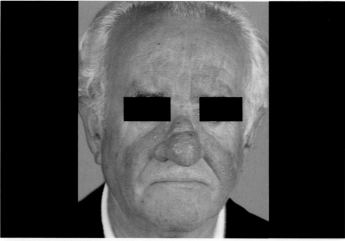

Figure 258. Rosacea. Extensive papular infiltrates in typical locations. There is beginning hyperplasia of the sebaceous glands of the nose. (Rhinophyma.)

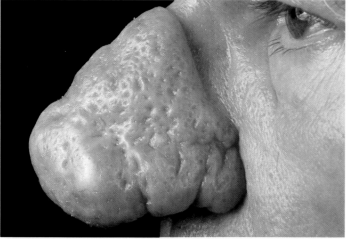

Figure 259. Rhinophyma. Distinct and sharply demarcated by pressure from the frame of the patient's glasses. Other symptoms of a facial rosacea are absent.

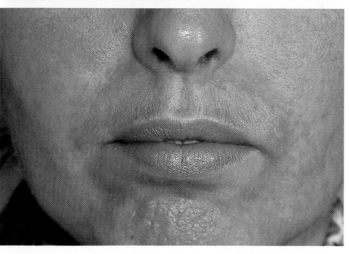

Figure 260. Perioral rosacea-like dermatitis. Infiltrates of small papules with typical sparing of the perioral area.

Rosacea and Rosacea-Like Dermatitis

Rosacea

Rosacea is a common chronic skin disease affecting mainly the face. It manifests itself in middle-aged persons and involves both sexes with the same frequency. The most disfiguring type, rhinophyma, occurs almost exclusively in men. The cause is unknown. Alcohol abuse, poorly balanced diet, or hyperseborrhea are associated with rosacea only in isolated cases.

Clinical Appearance

1. Persistent erythema, papules, and pustules as well as large inflammatory nodules and plaques can be present, depending on the severity of the disease. In contrast to acne, there are no comedones, even though the patient may have oily skin.
2. Areas of predilection are the cheeks, nose, forehead, and occasionally, the chin. Involvement is often in the shape of a "butterfly."
3. Involvement of the eyes with blepharitis, conjunctivitis, keratitis, and iridocyclitis can occur as a complication of rosacea.

Systemic Therapy

Rosacea requires systemic therapy only in severe cases.
1. Isotretinoin (R.60) in doses of 0.2 to 1 mg per kilogram of body weight for 10 to 16 weeks is recommended in Europe and has recently been approved for use in the United States.
2. Metronidazole, 250 mg per day for 10 days to a maximum of 20 days is helpful. Long-term therapy with metronidazole is contraindicated because of the risk of polyneuropathies and possible carcinogenic effects.
3. Long-term treatment with tetracyclines, as in acne (see p. 5), can be attempted but is often less effective.

Topical Therapy

The skin of rosacea patients becomes irritated very easily. Irritating substances or bases (salicylic acid, sulfur, fatty ointments) should be avoided.
1. The skin should be washed with detergents that have strong or weak defatting effects, depending on the type of skin.
2. Anti-inflammatory and antibacterial medications in a nonirritating base or benzoyl peroxide in a gel form 3 to 5% (R.24a) are often helpful.
3. Metronidazole is also effective when applied topically (1 to 2%).
4. Topical corticosteroids have no place in the treatment of rosacea. They can be effective over a short period of time, but the disease recurs after treatment is discontinued. Long-term therapy can result in "steroid damage" to the skin, which is very unpleasant in the face (erythema, telangiectasias, papules, hypertrichosis).
5. Hot drinks, exposure to steam, and alcohol consumption as well as intense sunlight exposure may increase the symptoms and should be avoided. Dietetic measures have no effect on rosacea.

Rosacea-Like Perioral Dermatitis

This disease occurs almost exclusively in women. So far, only fluorinated corticosteroids have been identified as causative substances.

Clinical Appearance

Pinhead-sized inflammatory papules appear on an erythematous base in the perioral region. A narrow band surrounding the lips is usually spared. The disease involves the surrounding skin only in severe cases.

Therapy

Corticosteroid therapy must be discontinued if the patient is on this medication. This is sometimes difficult because the skin changes usually increase in the beginning. The treatment should be supplemented with moist dressings (R.1) or lotions (R.20c). Ointments and creams with a strong lubricating effect must be avoided.

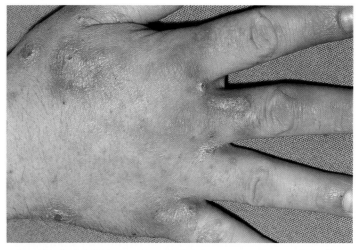

Figure 261. Scabies. Eczematization of the nodules and burrows mainly in the interdigital area.

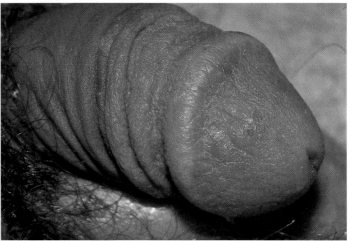

Figure 262. Scabies. Typical location of the nodules in a man: body and glans of the penis.

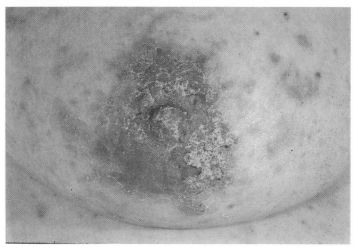

Figure 263. Scabies. Nonspecific eczematization. Typical location in a female patient: Region of the mamilla.

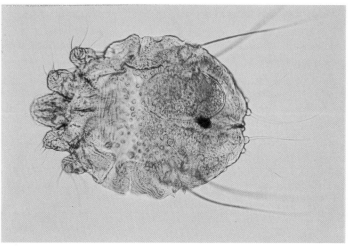

Figure 264. Scabies mite. Magnification 120×.

Scabies

The causative organism is the itch mite, Sarcoptes scabiei, *which is barely visible with the naked eye. Scabies occurs epidemically through close contact in families, nursing homes, orphanages, and so on. It is an infectious disease that affects all social levels and is not associated with poor body hygiene. It can also be transmitted by sexual intercourse, and in these cases, the diagnostic workup should include other sexually transmitted diseases.*

The disease is recognized by the burrows and papules that the female mite makes to deposit her eggs. These are always found in typical locations and are characterized by inflammatory reactions, formation of yellow crusts, weeping, pain, and marked pruritus. The diagnosis is confirmed by the demonstration of the causative organisms. The burrows are located and the mites removed with an injection needle. This can be troublesome but is desirable to establish the diagnosis. The incubation period is approximately 3 weeks. It is important to identify the source and treat all contact persons.

Clinical Appearance

1. Skin-colored or reddened, pinhead-sized papules or raised burrows several millimeters to 1 cm long are often visible. Eczematous eruptions with punctate erosions, crusts, and scales predominate, as well as secondary scratch marks.
2. These frequently uncharacteristic changes are located chiefly in the fingerwebs and the perimamillar and genital regions. The axillary folds, umbilical area, and buttocks are often involved.
3. Of diagnostic significance are pinhead-to pea-sized nodules on the shaft of the penis in men and in the mamillary region in women. In adults, the face and scalp as well as palms and soles are practically never involved. In children, vesicular eruptions are frequently seen on palms and soles.
4. Intensive itching, which is worse at night, as well as other infected cases in the environment, are additional important diagnostic clues.
5. Infection with Norwegian scabies or crusted scabies is characterized by the formation of heavy crusts on erythematous skin. It occurs mainly in persons with impaired immunity. Contrary to ordinary scabies, these crusts are heavily infested with mites and are very contagious. They are often the source of scabies epidemics in hospitals and nursing homes.

Therapy

1. An antiparasitic drug (lindane, benzyl benzoate, or crotamiton [R.38]) should be used on the skin from neck to toes daily for 3 days.

   The medication is applied at bedtime, and a bath should be taken in the morning to remove the drug. Bed sheets and clothing should be changed. In children, the drug is absorbed more readily, and its toxicity may be a hazard. Treatment in children should therefore be limited to one side or one quadrant for only a few hours at a time. Lindane should not be used during pregnancy; benzyl benzoate should be used instead (consult package insert).
2. Bed sheets or clothing used during the 2 days before treatment should be boiled or aired for 5 to 7 days to avoid reinfestation with mites that develop from the eggs. The mite can survive only 12 to 24 hours away from human skin.
3. Pruritus as well as eczematous lesions and postscabious papules can persist for several days or weeks after the mites have been killed. Application of corticosteroid creams (R.36a, c) is helpful.
4. Antihistamines (R.56, R.57) may be indicated for severe pruritus.
5. All infected persons must be treated to avoid reinfections (ping-pong infections).

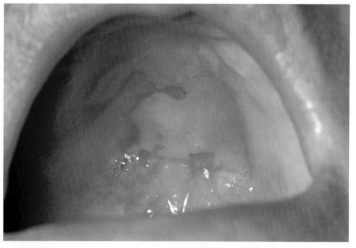

Figure 265. Stomatitis. Erythemata and erosions that are partly covered with fibrin.

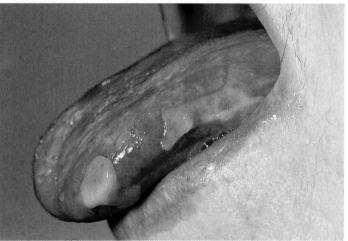

Figure 266. Drug-induced erosive-ulcerative stomatitis. The tongue is involved with fibrin-covered erosions.

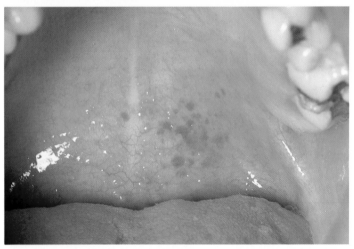

Figure 267. Herpangina Zahorsky. Vesicles on hard and soft palate are arranged unilaterally and in groups. The vesicles in this case have become hemorrhagic.

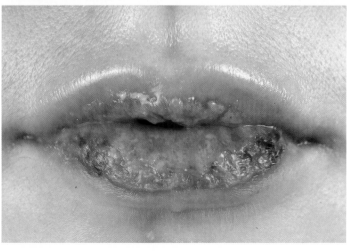

Figure 268. Stomatitis as part of an erythema multiforme. Typical crust formation on both lips.

Stomatitis, Inflammation of the Oral Mucosa

Stomatitis is an inflammation of the entire oral mucosa or major parts of it. It is only a symptom and requires further diagnostic clarification. Recurrent aphthae (see p. 7) are not associated with stomatitis. Stomatitis is usually a self-limited disease that develops to its full-blown appearance within 1 week and then subsides within 2 to 3 weeks. Stomatitis can appear as part of a viral disease, an undesired drug reaction, or an erythema multiforme. It can also be caused by bacterial infections (pyogenic gingivostomatitis), or it may be due to other permanent or transient immunosuppressive disorders such as leukemia and debilitating systemic diseases or to xerostomia.

Clinical Appearance

1. Erosions, fibrinous coatings, ulcers, and foul-smelling detritus are present in the anterior or the entire oral mucosa. Ulcers of the oral mucosa nearly always heal without scars, in contrast to the skin, where they do leave scars.
2. The gingiva is often involved in the form of gingivitis or gingivostomatitis.
3. The lesions cause pain with chewing, speaking, and even at rest. Not infrequently the patients also complain of an unpleasant, often metallic, taste (parageusia).
4. With severe stomatitis, there are blood coagula in the mouth and hemorrhagic crusts on the lips, especially when stomatitis is part of erythema multiforme.
5. Generalized symptoms such as weakness and indisposition are usually caused by the underlying disease and not by the stomatitis.

Therapy

It is very important to clarify the cause of the stomatitis so that specific therapeutic measures can be directed against the underlying disease. Symptomatic treatment consists of the following measures:

1. Rinse frequently with lukewarm water.
2. The diet should be liquid initially and soft later.
3. Bedrest is the most important general measure for severe stomatitis.
4. Systemic corticosteroids are indicated only for severe stomatitis but not for infectious stomatitis, such as gingivostomatitis herpetica.

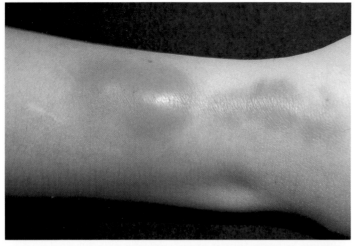

Figure 269. Acute thrombophlebitis. Chordlike, acute inflammatory infiltration along the course of a superficial vein.

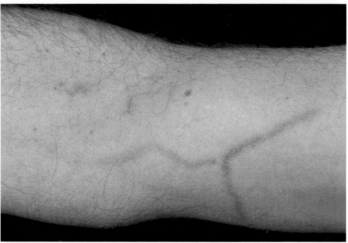

Figure 270. Pigmentation along the veins as sequel of a medication-induced thrombophlebitis.

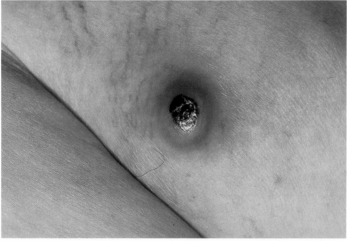

Figure 271. Ulcerated varix.

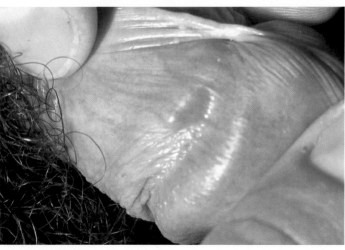

Figure 272. Phlebitis of the sulcus coronarius. Chordlike, occasionally painful induration of a vein in the sulcus coronarius.

Thrombophlebitis

Thrombophlebitis is a primary inflammation of the vein wall with secondary formation of a thrombus. Injury to the vein wall can be caused by injection of medications that irritate the vein wall, an indwelling venous catheter, or blunt trauma. Thrombophlebitis is also seen in patients with varicose veins and with certain generalized disorders such as Behçet's disease, typhoid fever and neoplastic diseases. Usually the thrombus adheres firmly to the vessel wall and, therefore embolization is extremely rare in thrombophlebitis.

Clinical Appearance

1. A chordlike, firm, very painful inflammatory infiltrate can be felt in the area of the affected vein with marked erythema of the overlying skin.
2. Iatrogenic thrombophlebitis is found almost exclusively on the arms. Otherwise, thrombophlebitis occurs much more frequently in the legs, in women more than in men.
3. A systemic reaction with fever, elevation of the sedimentation rate, leukocytosis, and generalized malaise is evident in many cases.
4. When massive inflammation is present, circumscribed necrosis can occur, with subsequent development of an ulcer (see p. 23).

Therapy

Systemic

1. Drugs that interfere with prostaglandin synthesis such as acetylsalicylic acid 1 to 3 g per day or indomethacin 50 to 100 mg per day are helpful. These medications have anti-inflammatory and analgesic effects.
2. Anticoagulant therapy may be necessary, but only in bedridden patients (low-dose heparin, rarely warfarin).

Topical

1. Cooling with alcohol dressings (R.1) can be helpful.
2. The patient should be made ambulatory with compression dressings.
3. When circumscribed nodular necrosis is present, the coagulum should be removed through a stab incision. This is then followed by a compression dressing.

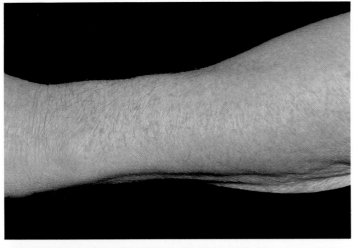

Figure 273. Dryness of the skin. Fine scaling in a patient with decreased turgor of the skin.

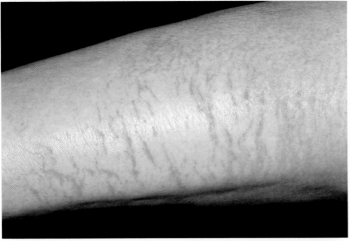

Figure 274. Dry skin with eczematization. Scaling with fissures and subsequent eczematization.

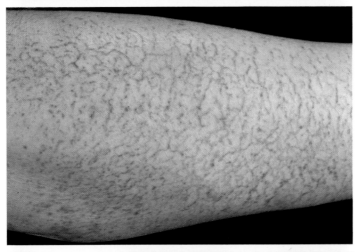

Figure 275. Eczema due to desiccation. Distinct hemorrhagic reticular eczema in fissures caused by the desiccation.

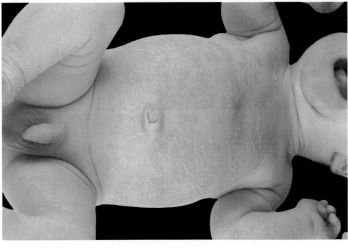

Figure 276. Ichthyosis vulgaris, so-called "fish skin disease." Marked scaling on trunk and extremities.

Dry Skin, Ichthyosis

Dryness of the Skin

A troublesome dryness of the skin is a frequent symptom with many causes. It is found especially in older persons with otherwise healthy skin in times of low humidity (winter, central heating), in people who wash and bathe too frequently, in patients with atopic dermatitis (see p. 47), and in patients with congenital ichthyosis. It can also occur as an undesirable side effect of some medications, such as spasmolytics with an atropine-like effect, synthetic retinoids (etretinate, isotretinoin), beta receptor blockers, H_2 receptor blockers (cimetidine, ranitidine), and tamoxifen.

Clinical Appearance

1. A disagreeable dryness of the skin is often a subjective symptom without visible skin changes. At a later time, fine scaling of the skin and pruritus often develop.
2. The dry skin of older people loses its turgor; the skin can be lifted up in folds and the folds return to their normal position much more slowly.
3. Scaling, superficial fissures, and pruritus develop as a result of the dryness, which may later lead to secondary eczematization or eczema formation with fissures (eczema craquelé). This is found especially on the lower legs, less often on the arms and trunks of older people.

Therapy

1. The dryness of the skin can be treated promptly and effectively by repeated topical application of water-containing fatty medications (R.31b). In patients with atopic dermatitis this should be done several times daily.
2. To condition the room climate, the room temperature must be lowered and the air humidified.

Ichthyosis, Fishskin

These are inherited disorders of keratinization that vary considerably in severity and are characterized by coarse, dry, and scaly skin.

Clinical Appearance

1. The skin is abnormally dry, with scaling that can be fine or coarse or rhomboid in shape or like reptile skin.
2. In the most common form, ichthyosis vulgaris, the flexor surfaces of the joints are spared; they are involved in the rare form of ichthyosis congenita.
3. The function of sebaceous and sweat glands is usually impaired, which can lead to thermoregulatory disturbances in hot weather and with intense physical activity.

Therapy

Causal therapy is not possible, but topical treatment can improve appearance and symptoms. Many patients find this long-term treatment too troublesome and apply the topical medication only sporadically or discontinue it altogether.

1. Urea-containing ointments (R.40b) are helpful for keratolysis and improve the water-retaining capacity of the skin.
2. Topical treatment can be supplemented by bath therapy with oily additives to lubricate the skin. A lubricating ointment (R.31b) should be applied after the bath to avoid excessive dehydration of the skin.
3. Severe cases may benefit from treatment with etretinate (R.59).
4. Occupations that cause degreasing of the skin (long-term contact with soaps, detergents, organic solvents, cement) should be avoided.

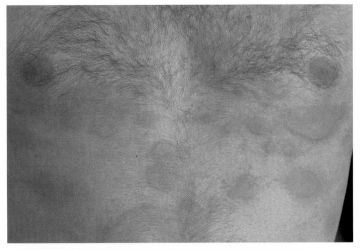

Figure 277. Urticaria. Coin-size reddened wheals on the trunk.

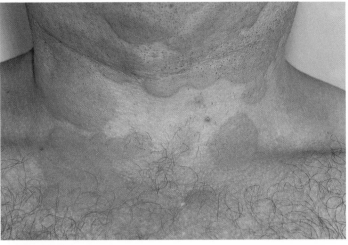

Figure 278. Urticaria. Transient wheals on neck and chest.

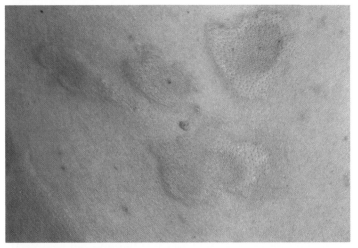

Figure 279. Urticaria. Wheals with raised margins. Pressure from the edema causes pallor of the raised margin.

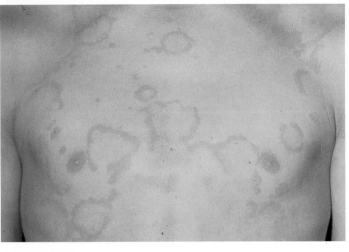

Figure 280. Urticaria. Wheals with raised margins. Coalescence of individual foci produces gyrated lesions.

Urticaria and Angioedema (Quincke's Edema)

Urticaria is characterized by transient wheals in the upper and middle layers of the skin. Angioedema (Quincke's edema) is an edema of the deep layers (subcutis). The causes of these polyetiologic symptoms are more or less identical. All factors that cause urticaria can also cause the much rarer angioedema. Both are reactions of the skin to either external and recognizable mechanisms or, much more often, internal and as yet unknown factors. Nonallergic causes are much more frequent than are allergic causes. Occasionally, urticaria or angioedema is accompanied by signs of shock: a drop in blood pressure, flushing, profuse perspiration, dyspnea, anxiety, tachycardia, and other symptoms.

Urticaria

A nonrecurring urticaria lasting not more than 4 to 6 weeks is called acute urticaria. Urticaria that lasts longer than 6 weeks or with recurrent attacks is termed chronic urticaria.

Causative factors of acute urticaria can be medications (especially the penicillins and cephalosporins as well as analgesics and x-ray contrast media), infections (virus infections such as hepatitis A, bacterial infections such as tonsillitis), the toxins of bee and wasp stings, foods, preservatives in drugs and food, and fruit acids. Such factors are found in approximately 50 per cent of all patients with acute urticaria. The causes of a chronic urticaria can be identified very rarely (in less than 5 per cent) even with a thorough workup. Chronic urticaria can be caused but only in rare instances, by traces of preservatives or food dyes or intestinal candidal infections.

Urticarial reactions may also be prompted by physical irritations (cold, heat, pressure, or sunlight) that can occur sporadically or have a familial tendency. Urticaria factitia (red urticarial dermographism) and finally cholinergic urticaria (minute urticarial foci after physical or emotional stress) are other expressions of urticaria.

Clinical Appearance

1. Transient, slightly elevated, round wheals without involvement of the epidermis are characteristic. The individual eruption usually persists 24 hours or less.
2. Marked edematous pressure makes the wheals appear whitish. They can have a raised margin and can coalesce into circinate lesions.
3. Pruritus is almost always present and usually severe.
4. All areas of the body may be involved, most frequently the trunk and extremities.
5. The special anatomic situations in penis, vulva, and oral mucosa do not permit wheals to develop; instead, edema occurs at these sites.

Therapy

It is important to determine the cause. Patients with chronic urticaria must be informed that it may not be possible to find the causes. Nevertheless, a thorough evaluation is indicated because an avoidable cause can sometimes be found.

Systemic

As long as no shock symptoms are present with acute urticaria, oral antihistamines (R.56, R.57) are sufficient. For chronic urticaria, cyproheptadine (Periactin) or hydroxyzine (Atarax, Vistaril) can be tried. Calcium is of little therapeutic value. Severe cases of acute urticaria should be treated with the measures described for angioedema (see later).

Shock symptoms must receive appropriate treatment depending on their severity (see p. 75).

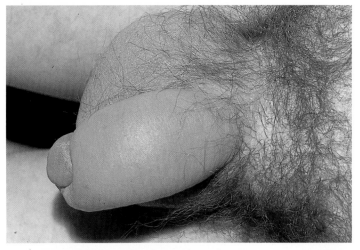

Figure 281. Urticaria. Diffuse edema of the penis. Due to the special texture of the connective tissue, wheals do not form at this site.

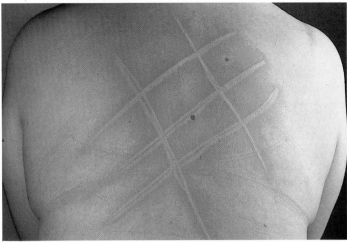

Figure 282. Urticarial dermographism. Wheals form following linear pressure to the skin.

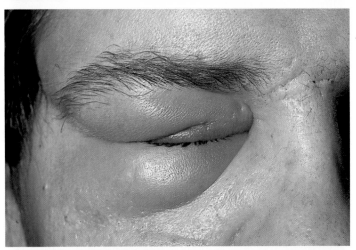

Figure 283. Angioedema. Unilateral massive transient edema, which in this patient is typically located in the lid area.

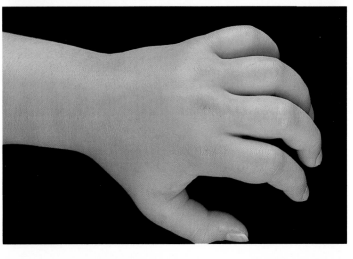

Figure 284. Hereditary angioedema with swelling of the hand.

Topical	Local treatment is rarely necessary and not effective. Antihistamines, locally administered, are not very effective; they can even cause an allergic or photoallergic contact dermatitis.
Prophylaxis	Many patients with chronic urticaria react to acetylsalicylic acid and other nonsteroidal analgesics or antirheumatic drugs with a new attack, occasionally with the symptoms of anaphylactoid shock. For this reason, analgesics should be used very selectively.

Angioedema (Quincke's Edema)

Angioedema can occur as an acute, one-time event or as a chronic recurrent problem simultaneously or alternating with urticaria. Chronic recurrent angioedema can also occur without urticaria. The possible causes of angioedema are just as manifold as those of urticaria and are more or less identical with them (see p. 141). Just as with chronic urticaria, there are recurrent angioedemas whose cause cannot be found even after thorough evaluation ("idiopathic angioedema"). The very rare hereditary angioedema is a separate entity and is characterized by familial occurrence of angioedemas of the skin, attacks of gastrointestinal pain, or edema attacks of internal organs. This disease is never associated with urticarial changes and is due to a $C\overline{1}$-inhibitor deficiency in the complement system. Very rarely, $C\overline{1}$-inhibitor deficiency and its clinical symptoms can be an acquired disorder.

Clinical Appearance

1. Skin-colored, mostly unilateral, swellings may persist for 2 to 5 days.
2. The periorbital region and lips are usually involved, but the swellings can occur in any part of the skin.
3. Subjectively, there is a feeling of tension and occasionally moderate pruritus and tension pain.
4. Swelling of the oral mucosa or swelling of internal organs can occur simultaneously or as an isolated finding.

Therapy

Hereditary angioedema must be excluded, because this disorder requires an entirely different therapeutic approach (see item 3 in the following). For the usual types of angioedema, determination of the cause is extremely important.

1. Angioedema can only be managed with systemic treatment. Intravenous antihistamines or intravenous corticosteroids are the drugs of choice.
2. For beginning laryngeal edema, the posterior wall of the pharynx must be sprayed with epinephrine; antihistamines, corticosteroids, or, if necessary, epinephrine (0.5 ml of a 1:1000 solution in 20 ml of 0.9% NaCl solution) may be given slowly intravenously. In extreme cases, intubation or tracheotomy may be necessary.
3. *Hereditary angioedema.* Substitution of the missing $C\overline{1}$-inhibitor ($C\overline{1}$ inactivator, Behring-Werke; Marburg, West Germany) must be made. In emergency cases, fresh frozen plasma, intravenous epinephrine, intubation, and tracheotomy are helpful. Corticosteroids alone are not effective, or at least not effective enough. These patients are best referred to a center with special experience in the treatment of this rare disorder.

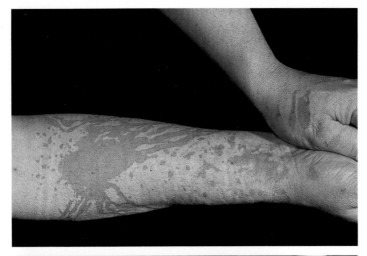

Figure 285. Hydrofluoric acid burn. Sharply demarcated erythema limited to the contact area.

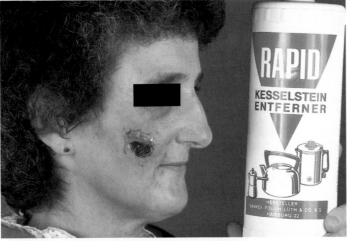

Figure 286. Acid burn caused by boiler scale remover containing amidosulfuric acid. Partially demarcated necrotic tissue on the right cheek.

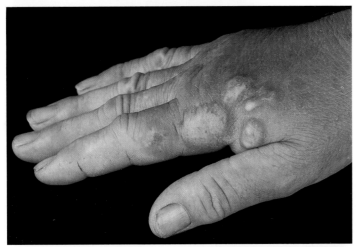

Figure 287. Burn caused by improper use of a plant protection agent. Erythema and formation of purulent bullae.

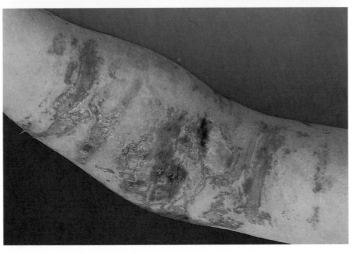

Figure 288. Burn caused by a solution used for pretzel making. Partly demarcated necroses and shallow ulcerations with beginning epithelial coverage.

Chemical Burns

A large number of industrial substances, as well as some household cleaners, can lead to contact injuries of the skin of varying degrees. The severity of the injury depends on how aggressive the substance was and how long it acted on the skin. Self-inflicted chemical burns (artifacts, see p. 9) and those occurring as a result of an unsuccessful suicide attempt are relatively few. The causative chemicals can act as oxydizing or reducing agents, as alkalis, as dehydrating substances, or as cell toxins.

Clinical Appearance

1. The injury is limited to the contact site, usually to an uncovered area of the body. Clinical signs can range from erythema, edema, or blister formation to the formation of white to black necroses, depending on the severity of the injury.
2. The extent of the injury cannot be estimated before demarcation of the necroses.
3. The amount of pain varies and depends largely on the damage to the sensory nerve fibers.

Therapy

1. The causative substance must be washed off immediately with copious amounts of fluid, preferably water. This is more important than wasting valuable time searching for a specific antidote.
2. Subsequent care does not differ significantly from that described for burns (see p. 147): removal of necrotic tissue with enzymatic ointments or by surgical debridement, followed by plastic coverage of the defect, with skin grafts where necessary.
3. Following emergency care of a chemical burn, one should always consult a poison control center regarding possible systemic effects of the substance or refer the patient to a center for further evaluation and treatment.
4. Tetanus prophylaxis is recommended.

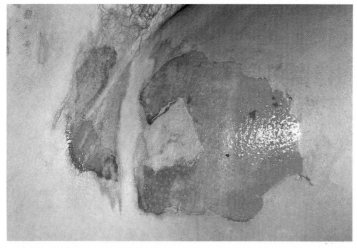

Figure 289. Scalding. Weeping erosions caused by hot steam.

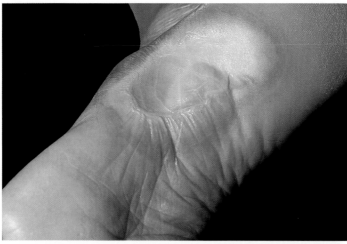

Figure 290. Third-degree burn. Whitish areas of necrosis with blister formation and marginal erythema caused by a hot water bottle in a patient with loss of sensation. The patient had complained about "cold feet" while under spinal anesthesia.

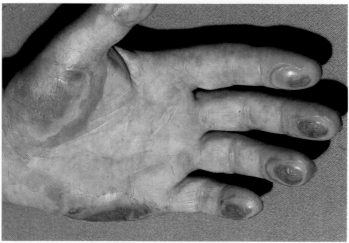

Figure 291. Second- and third-degree burns caused by a hot stove. Erosions and ulcers.

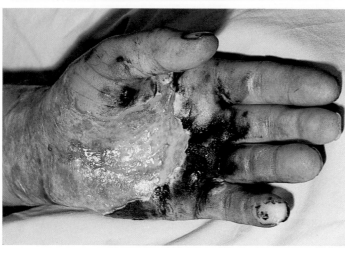

Figure 292. Tar burn.

Burns, Scalding

Burns are usually caused by industrial or household injuries, by traffic accidents, or during catastrophic events. They are classified according to the extent of tissue damage. Systemic effects of burns, especially on the cardiovascular system, immediately after injury as well as protracted toxic shock from absorption of toxins 3 to 5 days later must always be kept in mind. Burns are initially sterile, but bacterial contamination occurs rapidly, and infections, usually mixed infections, occur frequently. Infections in the hospital are caused chiefly by staphylococcus, streptococcus, and Pseudomonas aeruginosa. Systemic effects are due to not only the depth of the burn but also its extent. Burns of more than 9 per cent of the body surface always cause cardiovascular symptoms, which often predominate initially. Other possible systemic complications during the first few weeks include sepsis, anemia, transcutaneous loss of protein, and a derangement of the carbohydrate metabolism.

Clinical Appearance

First Degree Burn

Only the epidermis and the upper layers of the dermis are involved. Clinically, there is painful erythema and edema.

Second Degree Burn

In this stage, blisters and occasionally necroses of the epidermis develop.

Third Degree Burn

This causes deep tissue destruction with white necroses or charring. The nerve endings are often destroyed, sensitivity to pain is markedly reduced, or the injured areas are completely anesthetic.

Therapy

All third degree burns and extensive second degree burns must be treated in the hospital. Patients with severe burns should be referred to a burn center.

Before transporting the patient to the burn center, measures to combat shock must be initiated (IV line, infusion of an electrolyte solution, pain management), even if shock has not yet occurred.

For minor burns of first and second degree, the treatment is as follows.

Systemic

1. Pain should be treated. (Opiates may be necessary.)
2. Tetanus prophylaxis is recommended.
3. As soon as signs of wound infection appear, sensitivity of the organisms must be determined, followed by appropriate antibiotic therapy.

Topical

1. Cooling with cold water and moist dressings with disinfectant additives, especially aqueous silver nitrate solutions (R.2), are helpful.
2. In first and second degree burns, application of a corticosteroid cream (R.36b, c) for 2 to 3 days results in rapid improvement and pain relief.
3. Blisters should initially be left in place (protection against infection and mechanical insults, less pain). Tense blisters should be punctured under sterile conditions. Extensive erosions are covered with betadine ointment or Vaseline gauze.
4. Topical application of antibiotics or sulfonamides is not recommended because of possible contact allergy and because they promote resistance of the organisms.

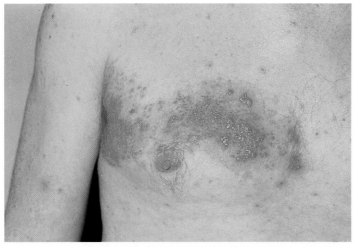

Figure 293. Herpes zoster. Segmental erythema with grouped blisters. Note the isolated blisters outside the segment (aberrant blisters).

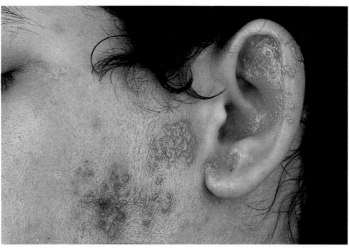

Figure 294. Herpes zoster in the segment supplied by *N. trigeminus*. The grouped vesicles are arranged in a strictly segmental fashion.

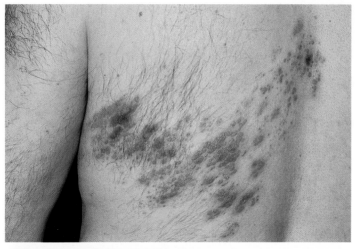

Figure 295. Herpes zoster in the thorax region with hemorrhagic vesicles.

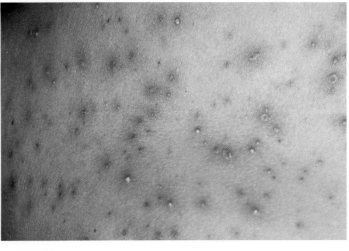

Figure 296. Disseminated herpes zoster. Dissemination of individual blisters over the entire skin in addition to the typical segmental involvement. The appearance resembles chickenpox.

Herpes Zoster, Shingles

Herpes zoster is the secondary manifestation of an infection with the varicella zoster virus. It can occur at any age but is much more common in older people. In the elderly, the course of the disease is more severe and frequently followed by prolonged and severe neuralgia. When herpes zoster occurs with Hodgkin's disease or other immunosuppressive diseases, the illness can run a life-threatening course (meningitis, encephalitis, sepsis). A patient who has severe involvement with blister formation on the entire skin (generalized herpes zoster) should always be evaluated for a malignant disease. A syntropy between the involved dermatome and diseases of the internal organs associated with the affected neural segment has often been suggested but has not been confirmed.

Clinical Appearance

1. The disease is characterized by groups of vesicles on an erythematous base that develop in batches. The vesicles are clear initially and then develop into pustules. In severe cases, they can become hemorrhagic or necrotic (hemorrhagic zoster, gangrenous zoster). The vesicles develop in one neural segment with occasional dissemination of individual vesicles over the entire skin (zoster varicellosus).
2. The zoster eruption is always unilateral and is limited to one (rarely several adjacent) neural segment. The first division of the trigeminal nerve and the thoracic region are involved most often. Lesions of the eye (conjunctivitis, iritis) entail the risk of permanent visual damage and require ophthalmologic care. Vesicles on the bridge and tip of the nose are indicative of eye involvement.
3. The skin eruptions are preceded and accompanied by pain in the segmental dermatome. In older patients, this pain can persist as a very troublesome neuralgia. In children, herpes zoster is often painless. Motor nerves can also be involved and result in paresis (disturbance of oculomotor function and visual accommodation—facial paresis). The regional lymph nodes are usually enlarged and tender.
4. Infection can occur with direct skin contact; patients with impaired immunity against varicella are also at risk.

Therapy

Systemic

Acyclovir has a virostatic effect. In mild cases, it is given orally; in more severe cases, intravenously (acyclovir 5 mg per kilogram of body weight 3 times daily). In immunocompromised patients, the course of the disease can be mitigated by varicella hyperimmune globulin given in the early phase of the disease (very expensive). In young patients and those with a mild course, there is no systemic therapy necessary.

Systemic symptomatic therapy is aimed mainly at pain relief. It must be kept in mind that a constant level of the analgesic drug should be maintained for adequate relief of pain, which means that the drug has to be given at regular intervals determined by its half-life. With this method, even severe pain can often be treated with relatively mild to moderate analgesics, such as paracetamole (acetaminophen), acetylsalicylic acid, or indomethacin, especially when they are combined with drugs that raise the pain threshold (thioridazine, carbamazepine). Severe pain that cannot be relieved with these measures may occasionally require the use of strong analgesics (tramadol or opiates). "Neurotropic vitamins" (B_1, B_6, B_{12}) have often been recommended for this disease, but their therapeutic effectiveness has never been proven. Systemic corticosteroids can be used as prophylaxis for postherpetic neuralgia; the possible side effects must be taken into account.

Topical

Moist compresses or painting with a zinc shake mixture can be helpful. In the early stage (stage of eruption), compresses with Burow's solution can be used to dry up the vesicles. Remnants of the vesicles are best removed with an antibiotic ointment.

Nerve blocks may be indicated for severe postherpetic neuralgia that cannot be relieved with other measures.

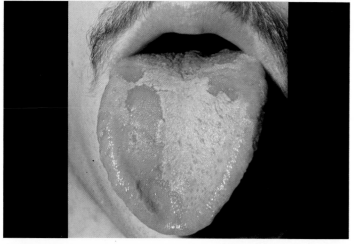

Figure 297. Lingua geographica (geographic tongue). Decreased keratinization of the filiform papillae of the tongue in round confluent areas. This is a rapidly changing harmless condition.

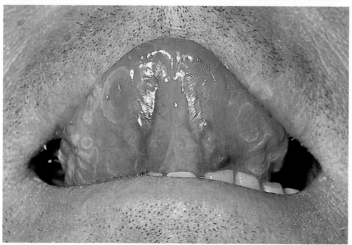

Figure 298. Lingua geographica (geographic tongue). Lesions with raised margins on the underside of the tongue.

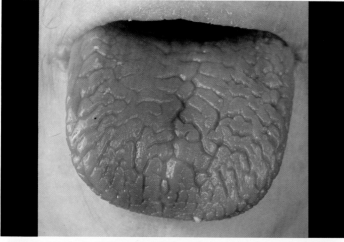

Figure 299. Lingua plicata.

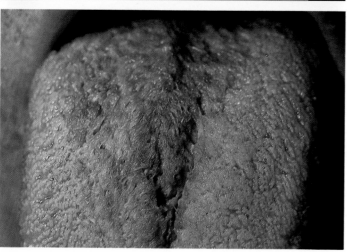

Figure 300. Lingua villosa nigra (black, hairy tongue). Elongation and brownish discoloration of the filiform papillae of the tongue extending anteriorly and laterally.

Disorders of the Tongue

The tongue is affected in the course of many generalized diseases, especially as part of the aphthous or erosive ulcerative stomatitis of many viral diseases. There are other disorders of the tongue that are harmless changes but can often disquiet the patients who are affected with them.

Lingua Geographica

These are transitory migrant plaques whose appearance changes rapidly. They are due to focal hypokeratinization of the filiform papillae.

Clinical Appearance

1. The disorder is characterized by one or several patches that are darker than the normal surface of the tongue and occasionally have a white or yellow margin.
2. The patches develop and grow rapidly within a few days to form gyrate lesions.
3. Usually only the dorsal surface of the tongue and especially the marginal areas are involved. The undersurface and the oral mucosa are rarely affected.
4. Subjective symptoms are minimal: There may be mild tenderness, increased by the ingestion of sour food.

Therapy

The patient should be informed that the condition is harmless. No effective treatment is available.

Lingua Plicata, Fissured Tongue

The physiologic grooves of the tongue are enlarged, usually a harmless congenital condition. In rare instances, it can be associated with chronic swelling of the lips and facial paresis (Melkersson-Rosenthal syndrome).

Clinical Appearance

1. There are deep grooves on the dorsal surface of the tongue that are often shaped like the veins of a leaf. Erosions develop in the depth of the grooves from lack of the rinsing and cleansing action of the saliva.
2. The condition is rarely painful, except when spicy food is eaten.

Therapy

Treatment is necessary only for deep erosions, for which disinfectant mouthwashes are useful.

Lingua Villosa Nigra, Black Hairy Tongue

The condition is due to increased keratinization of the filiform papillae. The dark color is also caused by embedded food remnants and chromogenic bacteria. Lingua villosa nigra often occurs without a recognizable cause. Occasionally, it can develop after treatment with broad-spectrum antibiotics or rarely after treatment with corticosteroids or mouth washing with H_2O_2.

Clinical Appearance

1. Black or greenish-brown discoloration of the elongated filiform papillae is characteristic. The changes begin at the base of the tongue and spread anteriorly and laterally, forming a triangular field pointing forward.
2. Usually, there are no subjective symptoms.

Therapy

Treatment is not very promising. Lingua villosa nigra regresses spontaneously after several weeks or months or occasionally after several years.

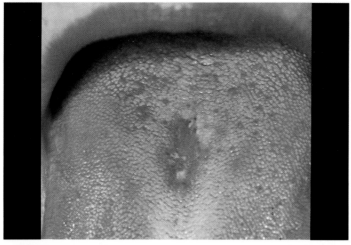

Figure 301. Median rhomboid glossitis (glossitis rhombica mediana). Rhomboid depression of the posterior section of the tongue medially and dorsally.

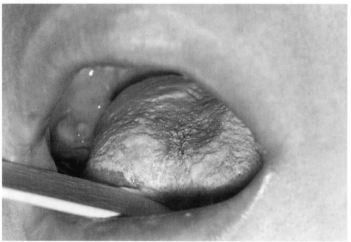

Figure 302. Increased coating of the tongue in a patient with erosive stomatitis and cheilitis.

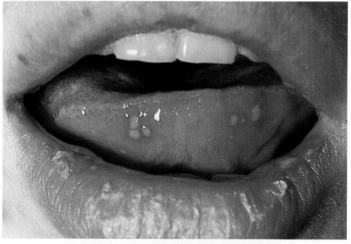

Figure 303. Aphthae of the tongue in a patient with viral aphthoid stomatitis.

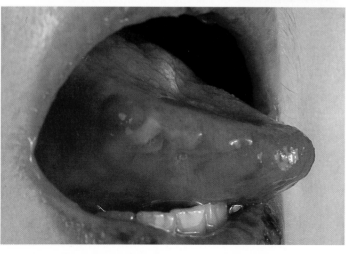

Figure 304. Erosive-ulcerative glossitis in a patient with drug-induced inflammation of the oral mucous membrane.

Glossitis Rhomboidea Mediana

This is a depression or elevation in the midline of the tongue that usually appears in midlife or old age. It is assumed that the cause of the condition is a developmental defect, a persisting tuberculum impar.

Clinical Appearance

1. A rhomboid smooth area approximately 1 by 2 cm, without papillae, located in the long axis of the tongue is characteristic. It can be either depressed or elevated in an irregular, nodular fashion. The area can develop a leukoplakia-like aspect secondarily.
2. The changes are located in the midline at the junction between the posterior and middle third of the tongue.
3. There are no subjective symptoms. The patients usually consult a physician because they fear they have cancer.

Therapy

No effective treatment exists for this harmless developmental anomaly. In some cases, the condition responds to antimycotic therapy (e.g., nystatin suspension), probably because of secondary infection with *Candida albicans*.

Increased Coating of the Tongue

"Coating" of the tongue appears as a whitish discoloration of the dorsal surface. It is due to a transient increase in keratinization of the filiform papillae and can be caused by inflammatory changes or by decreased desquamation. Increased coating of the tongue is seen in conditions with high fever, such as upper respiratory infections. Desquamation is decreased when no solid food is eaten, especially in patients on parenteral feeding. The increased coating normally seen in the morning is caused by reduced desquamation due to diminished movements of the tongue during sleep. Coating is found more in the posterior parts of the tongue because movement, and thus abrasion, is less pronounced than it is on the tip or margins of the tongue.

Part II

Sexually Transmitted Diseases and Nonvenereal Genital Diseases

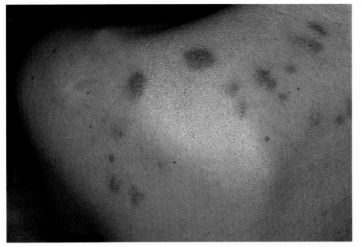

Figure 305. Kaposi's sarcoma in a patient with AIDS. Disseminated red-brown tumors on the shoulder.

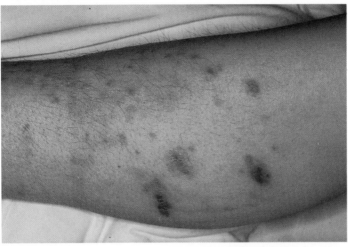

Figure 306. Kaposi's sarcoma in a patient with AIDS. Multiple brown-red or blue-red angiosarcomas of the calf.

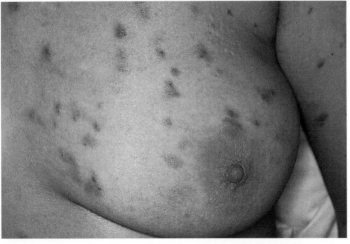

Figure 307. Kaposi's sarcoma in AIDS simulating prurigo.

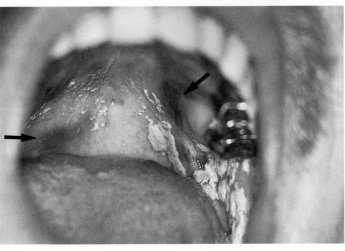

Figure 308. AIDS—Kaposi's sarcomas (→) and thick white coatings caused by marked candidiasis.

AIDS

At the present time, AIDS (acquired immune deficiency syndrome) has become a common disease, and an increase of these cases must be expected. Knowledge of the symptomatology, as well as of the skin changes, is therefore absolutely necessary for the practicing physician. The disease occurs mainly in male homosexuals, but it is seen in other men, women, and children. It is caused by retrovirus HIV, which can survive outside the body for only a short time. The infection is transmitted by body tissue containing the causative organisms, primarily sperm and blood, that enters the body through usually minor injuries (e.g., mucosal tears).

The organism is transmitted through homosexual intercourse (where minor injuries occur frequently) or bisexual intercourse, in drug addicts through the use of contaminated injection needles, and, in rare instances, through transfusion of blood from infected donors. At high risk are promiscuous male homosexuals, bisexual males who change their partners frequently, heterosexual partners of infected persons, persons addicted to intravenously administered drugs, hemophiliacs, and newborn babies of infected mothers. Exact immunologic workup is elaborate and should be done at an AIDS clinic. The prognosis for the disease is poor; most patients with manifest symptoms of AIDS die within a few years.

Clinical Appearance

1. Symptoms of the acute infection are fever, swelling of the lymph nodes, and discrete exanthema several weeks after exposure to the virus. These symptoms are observed only rarely. The symptom-free latent phase can last from 2 months to 6 years. Lymphadenopathy syndrome (LAS) is present when patients with confirmed HIV infection exhibit enlarged lymph nodes in at least two parts of the body that are regionally not connected for 3 or more months. Other symptoms that can occur individually or in combination are persistent or intermittent fever, fatigue, loss of appetite, weight loss (more than 10 per cent without recognizable cause), nausea, diarrhea of more than 1 week's duration, as well as increased sweating, night sweats, and varying skin infections. This stage can last for several months or years.

2. As long as the immune system is suppressed, life-threatening infections, such as pneumonia caused by *Pneumocystis carinii* and persistent infections with cytomegalovirus, herpes simplex virus, and toxoplasma, occur frequently. Candidal infections of skin and oral mucosa resistant to therapy are often found, especially with cheilitis angularis (perlèche, see p. 109).

3. Kaposi's sarcoma of the skin, an angiosarcoma, is one of the symptoms of advanced AIDS. The clinical features include disseminated purple to dark red or blue to brownish red vascular tumors that are often oval and are oriented along the creases of the skin. Occasionally, they are found on the mucous membranes of mouth, nose, eyes, and rectum.

4. Infectious skin diseases such as folliculitis, abscesses, impetigo, syphilis, tuberculosis, candidiasis, other fungal diseases, and common warts are common in AIDS patients. Other skin diseases seen in AIDS are seborrheic dermatitis and papular eruptions.

Therapy

Effective causal therapy does not exist at the present time. Some patients seem to benefit from azidodeoxythymidine. Symptomatic treatment of opportunistic infections is necessary.

Prophylaxis

No blood donations should be accepted from members of risk groups. Frequent change of sexual partners should be avoided. Condoms and other protective measures must be used. Sexual partners, attending physicians, and dentists (risk of infection during bloody procedures) must be informed of positive results of HIV tests. Members of the health professions must observe the same guidelines for prophylaxis against infection as those being taken against hepatitis B.

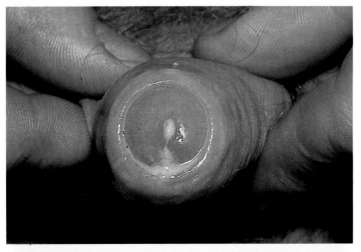

Figure 309. Typical appearance of acute gonorrhea with purulent discharge in a man.

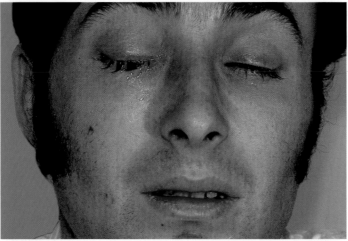

Figure 310. Gonoblennorrhea. Gonorrheic conjunctivitis caused by contact infection.

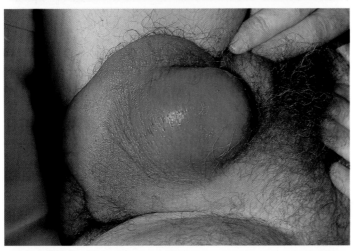

Figure 311. Gonorrhea. Extensive inflammatory conglomerate tumor in the area of the left adnexae caused by gonorrheic orchiepididymitis.

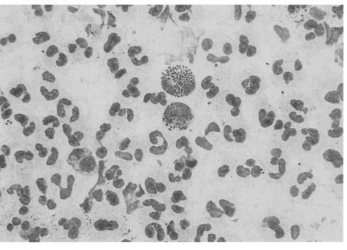

Figure 312. *Neisseria gonorrhoeae*. Typical appearance of intracellular organisms in a methylene blue–stained smear (630×).

Gonorrhea

Gonorrhea is one of the most common bacterial infectious diseases. Transmission is possible only through sexual intercourse because of the organism's high sensitivity to oxygen and desiccation. Changes in sexual and recreational behavior allow more and more penicillin- and spectinomycin-resistant organisms to be introduced from Southeast Asia. A smear stained with a relatively simple methylene blue or Gram's stain can be used as a screening test. The organisms appear as gram-negative diplococci usually located within leukocytes. The diagnostic value of this method is not very specific because of the similar morphology of other Neisseria. *It is not sensitive enough in chronic gonorrhea because of the relative paucity of organisms. In persons who change their sexual partners frequently, and in patients suspected of having chronic gonorrhea, the organisms should be identified by culture with subsequent sensitivity studies. A smear can be taken in the physician's office and mailed to a laboratory in an appropriate medium.*

Clinical Appearance

Gonorrhea in the Male

1. Following an incubation period of 3 (1 to 14) days, an acute inflammation of the anterior parts of the urethra occurs with a purulent discharge that is increased in the morning.
2. The patient complains of marked burning with urination.
3. During the subsequent course of the disease, the posterior urethra, the prostate (chronic prostatitis), and the epididymis (acute epididymitis) may become involved. The patient then complains of severe pain, swelling, and generalized malaise.
4. Homosexuals may develop rectal or pharyngeal infections with *Neisseria*.

Gonorrhea in the Female

Clinical manifestations of the disease differ, depending on the location of the infection.
1. Gonorrheal urethritis shows the clinical signs of acute urethritis (dysuria, frequency, and so on).
2. Cervicitis may be present. There is increased vaginal discharge but no other symptoms.
3. Infection of Bartholin's glands with abscess formation is often accompanied by marked swelling of the external genitals, erythema, and pain.
4. Rectal or pharyngeal infections are also possible.
5. Chronic infection of the fallopian tubes can lead to adhesions in the tubes and subsequent sterility.
6. Rarely, a septic infection can occur with chills, high fever, arthralgia, and metastatic skin lesions (hemorrhagic pustules).

Therapy

1. Penicillin (R.45), 4 million units intramuscularly (i.m.) for 3 days, or a one-time dose of 4.8 million units of penicillin i.m. plus 1 g probenecid by mouth is recommended. As an alternative to painful i.m. injections, one oral dose of 3 g of amoxicillin (R.46) in combination with 1 g of probenecid can be given.
2. Spectinomycin (R.51), 2 g i.m. for men, 4 g i.m. for women, is used for infections with organisms resistant to penicillin and in patients allergic to penicillin.
3. For penicillin-resistant organisms, cephalosporins can be used, for instance 1 g cephtriaxon (Rocephin) i.m. one time. Tetracyclines require a longer treatment period (2 g daily for 5 to 7 days).
4. The patients should always be evaluated for other venereal diseases, especially AIDS and syphilis, even after a confirmed diagnosis of gonorrhea.
5. The diagnosis "gonorrhea resistant to treatment" can occasionally mask an infection with *Chlamydia*, *Mycoplasma*, or *Trichomonas*.
6. The legal reporting regulations must be observed.

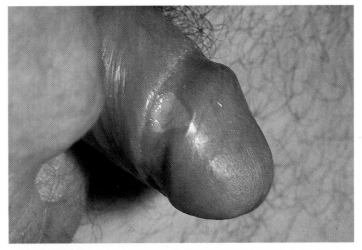

Figure 313. Syphilis I. Primary lesion. Firm, fibrin-covered ulcer with reddened margin.

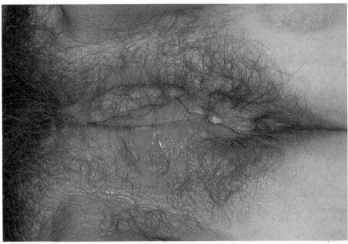

Figure 314. Syphilis I. Primary lesion. Ulcer with ham-colored floor.

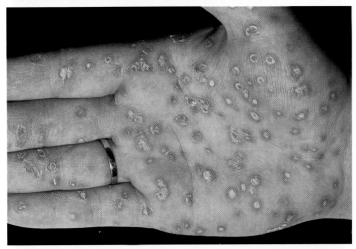

Figure 315. Syphilis II. Lenticular, psoriasiform, scaling papules on the palm of the hand.

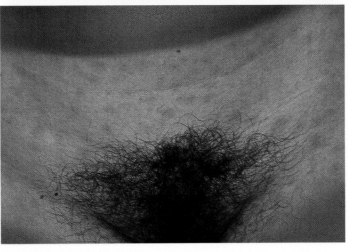

Figure 316. Syphilis II. Pale, macular exanthema, in this case, visible only in nontanned areas. So-called roseola syphilitica.

Syphilis

Syphilis is still one of the most significant and most common venereal diseases. It is transmitted most often by sexual intercourse. Infection is also possible through contact with secretions and blood that contain organisms. During pregnancy, an infected mother can transmit the disease to her fetus. Untreated syphilis can lead to death during the late stages. The morphology of syphilitic skin changes is manifold, especially in the secondary stage, and should always be considered in the differential diagnosis of exanthematous skin changes together with viral exanthems and drug eruptions. Diagnostic workup for syphilis should include clinical appearance, identification of the causative organisms (Treponema pallidum) in the tissue fluid, and the demonstration of specific antibodies with different serologic methods (TPHA test, VDRL test, FTA test). At least two of these three diagnostic tests must be positive to confirm a diagnosis of syphilis.

The course of the disease can be divided into four stages.

Primary Stage: Stage of the primary lesion (hard chancre) with subsequent swelling of the regional lymph nodes.

Secondary Stage: Stage of generalization. This stage begins approximately 7 weeks after infection and lasts approximately 2 years.

Tertiary Stage: So-called organ syphilis, occurs after 3 to 10 years.

Neurosyphilis: Tabes dorsalis and general paralysis manifest themselves after 15 to 30 years.

Clinical Appearance

Primary Syphilis

1. A small, painless nodule develops at the site of inoculation 10 to 14 days after infection. This nodule is often overlooked. It evolves into the primary lesion, an eroded, painless, weeping, indurated ulcer. The causative organisms can usually be demonstrated by darkfield examination in the serum of the primary lesion.
2. Since the disease is transmitted by sexual intercourse, approximately 90 per cent of all syphilitic primary lesions are found in the genital area, in men on the glans penis, on the sulcus coronarius, or on the shaft of the penis. In women, primary lesions are observed less frequently. They usually appear on the labia majora or minora or on the cervix. Depending on the patient's sexual practices, perianal or oral chancres can also be found.
3. The accompanying unilateral (rarely bilateral) painless enlargement of the lymph nodes that occurs approximately 1 week after the primary lesion is typical for the disease.

Secondary Stage

1. Skin manifestations of the secondary stage appear approximately 6 to 12 weeks after the infection. At this time, the chancre has often not healed yet or is visible as a fresh scar. The early symptoms of the secondary stage consist of a pale macular exanthem located primarily on the trunk (roseola syphilitica). Later, new crops of eruptions appear; the macular lesions gradually change into papules. In the genital and perianal regions as well as other moist areas (e.g., interdigital webs of the toes), these pale red to dark red papules may form weeping lesions (condylomata lata). The secretions of these lesions are full of treponemes and are highly infectious. Palms and soles are often affected; the exanthem in these areas frequently resembles psoriasis. Often hair loss occurs in a diffuse, spotty distribution (moth-eaten).
2. In immunosuppressed patients, a so-called lues maligna can develop, with weeping, erosive-ulcerative destructive infiltrates covered with crusts.
3. Exanthematous lesions on the oral mucosa show rapid ulcerative destruction (plaques muqueuses).
4. Generalized indurated and painless swelling of the lymph nodes is present during the secondary stage of syphilis.
5. Systemic manifestations can be transient fever, shin pain, pharyngitis, and hepatitis.

161

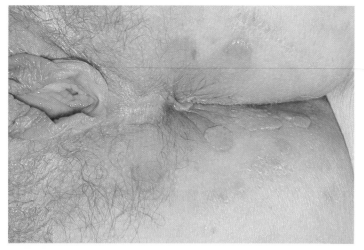

Figure 317. Syphilis II. Condylomata lata. Wide, soft, superficially weeping, highly infectious papules.

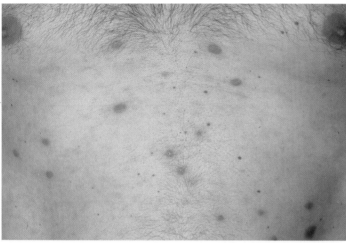

Figure 318. Syphilis II. Lenticular, brownish papules and pale brownish, macular exanthema.

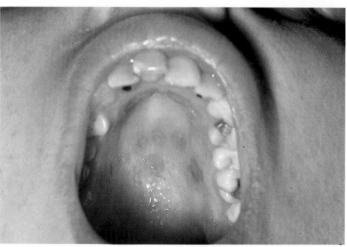

Figure 319. Syphilis II. Involvement of the mucous membrane of the mouth. Sharply demarcated erosions on the hard palate.

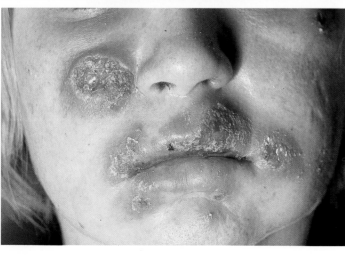

Figure 320. Syphilis II. So-called lues maligna. Pronounced inflammatory reaction with crusty and weeping infiltrates.

Tertiary Syphilis	Tertiary syphilis is seen very rarely today. This stage is characterized by circumscribed serpiginous foci that consist of small individual nodules and continue to enlarge peripherally (tuberoserpiginous syphilid). Growth continues over months or even years. Circumscribed granulomas (gummas) that develop subcutaneously frequently become necrotic with central ulceration or perforation (for instance on the hard palate). Cardiovascular syphilis can represent a vital danger to the patient with the development of an aortic aneurysm.

Tertiary Syphilis

Tertiary syphilis is seen very rarely today. This stage is characterized by circumscribed serpiginous foci that consist of small individual nodules and continue to enlarge peripherally (tuberoserpiginous syphilid). Growth continues over months or even years. Circumscribed granulomas (gummas) that develop subcutaneously frequently become necrotic with central ulceration or perforation (for instance on the hard palate). Cardiovascular syphilis can represent a vital danger to the patient with the development of an aortic aneurysm.

Neurosyphilis

Tabes dorsalis and general paralysis are hardly known to the general practitioner today. A positive history, positive serologic reaction in connection with neurologic or psychiatric symptoms (ataxia, loss of depth perception, and absent patellar and Achilles tendon reflexes) are indicative of tabes dorsalis. Psychiatric disorders, such as progressive dementia, manic depressive symptoms, or paranoia and hallucinations, should make one think of general paralysis. The patient should be referred to a neurologist or a psychiatrist for confirmation of the diagnosis.

Therapy

The drug of choice is penicillin G. Doses recommended by the Centers for Disease Control (CDC) are usually slightly lower than those used in Europe. (European doses will appear in parentheses.)

1. For early syphilis (primary and secondary stages until 1 year post infection), benzathine penicillin G, 2.4 million units total, i.m., in a single dose (in Europe, clemizole penicillin [megacillin] 1,000,000 I.U. i.m. daily for 18 days) is recommended.
2. As an alternative in patients allergic to penicillin, tetracycline hydrochloride 500 mg by mouth (p.o.) every 6 hours for 15 days or erythromycin 500 mg p.o. every 4 hours for 15 days can be given.
3. For syphilis of more than 1 year's duration the following is recommended: benzathine penicillin G, 2.4 million units, i.m. once a week for 3 successive weeks (7.2 million units total) (in Europe, clemizole penicillin [megacillin] 1,000,000 I.U. i.m. daily for 21 days; 500 mg p.o. every 6 hours for 30 days or erythromycin 500 mg p.o. every 6 hours for 30 days.
4. Failures with this therapeutic regimen are extremely rare and are usually reinfections.
5. After termination of treatment, serologic checkups are necessary at regular intervals to verify success of treatment: in early syphilis, every 3 months for 1 year, in late syphilis every 3 months for at least 3 years. *Treponema*-specific IgG antibodies are usually present for the remainder of the patient's life; they can be demonstrated with the FTA and TPHA tests. These antibodies do not protect against reinfection. IgM FTA and VDRL test titers decrease significantly with therapy and can even become negative.
6. When treating patients with syphilis, public health regulations, including reporting, must be observed.

Careful documentation of patient data, physical findings, and therapeutic measures and their results is absolutely necessary. It is also important to advise the patient that he or she must abstain from sexual relations until treatment is completed and that he or she must inform any sexual partners, who should seek medical help.

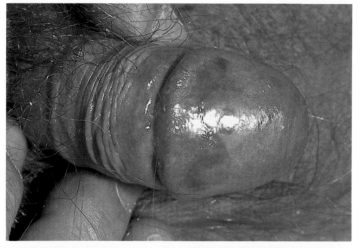

Figure 321. Balanitis simplex. Acute inflammation with erythematous weeping lesions on glans penis and prepuce.

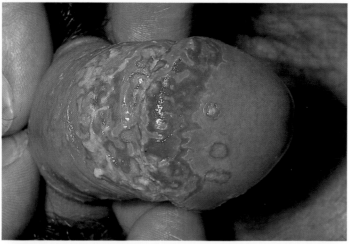

Figure 322. Genital herpes. Painful erosions that are often arranged in a clover leaf fashion as a sequel of the pre-existing vesicles.

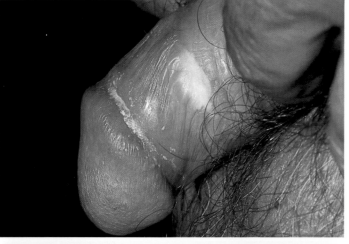

Figure 323. Balanitis xerotica obliterans. Atrophic changes with erosions and leukoplakia.

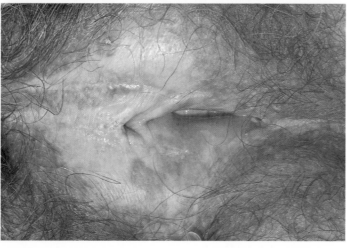

Figure 324. Lichen sclerosus et atrophicus. Extensive atrophy of the external female genital organs. Distinct whitening of the atrophic areas.

Nonvenereal Genital Diseases

Balanitis

Balanitis is an inflammation of the glans penis; balanoposthitis is an inflammation of the glans penis with involvement of the internal mucous lining of the prepuce. The anatomic relationships of the preputial space predispose to inflammation from bacteria, yeast, or irritating agents (spermicide aphrodisiacs, medications), especially when genital hygiene is either poor or excessive. Generalized infections, excessive coffee consumption, and insufficient bedrest can also promote an acute balanitis.

Clinical Appearance
1. Initially, there is only erythema and foul-smelling watery secretion.
2. Longer-lasting inflammations or phimosis can lead to retention of secretions and maceration followed by ulceration with purulent discharge.
3. A secondary candidiasis develops frequently.
4. Chronic balanitis is often seen in patients with diabetes mellitus.

Therapy
1. The penis should be soaked in disinfectant solutions or detergents ($KMnO_4$ solution 1:10,000).
2. Moist dressings, provided the prepuce can be reduced, are helpful. Otherwise, irrigate the preputial space with a bulbous cannular syringe.
3. A bland zinc oxide paste is effective (R.27, R.28), applied subsequent to an antimycotic solution (R.14c).
4. The causes must be eliminated to avoid a recurrence.

Vulvovaginitis

Acute vulvovaginitis is usually infectious (gonorrhea, herpes, candidiasis, trichomoniasis, syphilis). It can also be caused by a contact dermatitis. Chronic vulvovaginitis is frequently due to candidiasis in patients with diabetes mellitus.

Clinical Appearance
1. Inflammatory erythema and swelling of the external genitals with erosions and increased vaginal discharge are characteristic. The vaginal mucosa is often involved.
2. The main subjective symptom is pruritus, but the patients can occasionally complain of moderate to severe pain.

Therapy
The cause should be eliminated if at all possible. Symptomatic treatment includes sitzbaths with disinfectant solutions (R.4), moist compresses (R.1), zinc oil or zinc lotion (R.20), and dabbing with gentian violet solution (0.1 to 0.5% watery solution). Ointments should be avoided; they frequently cause an exacerbation.

Lichen Sclerosus et Atrophicus, Balanitis Xerotica Obliterans

Lichen sclerosus et atrophicus is a connective tissue disease affecting mainly the genitals. It leads to a progressive atrophy of the vulva in women or increasing phimosis and atrophy of the prepuce and glans penis in men (balanitis xerotica obliterans). The advanced stage may predipose to leukoplakia (see p. 213), a precancerous lesion.

Clinical Appearance
1. White atrophic lesions with parchment-like shriveling of the skin are characteristic. Not infrequently, one also sees small keratotic flakes associated with the follicles. Widespread atrophy of the external genitals develops with advancing disease.

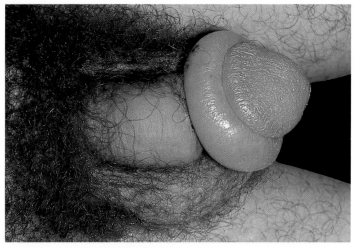

Figure 325. Paraphimosis (appearance of a "Spanish collar"). Massive circular edema of the foreskin peripheral to the constriction band of a phimotic prepuce.

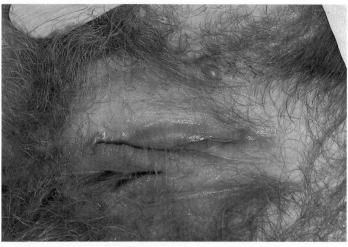

Figure 326. Varices of the vulva.

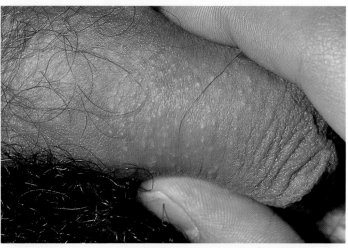

Figure 327. Ectopic sebaceous glands on the body of the penis, a frequently seen harmless condition.

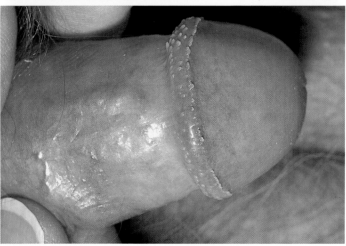

Figure 328. Hirsuties papillaris penis. Filiform papillomata on the junction between glans penis and sulcus coronarius. Harmless variation of the norm.

2. The vulva is affected in women, the prepuce and glans penis in men.
3. The disorder can occasionally cause obliteration of the urethral orifice with severe impairment of urination.
4. Often there is severe pruritus, and the patient's constant scratching causes inflammation with further increase of pruritus.

Therapy

A causal therapy does not exist. Marked phimosis or severe urethral stenosis must be treated surgically. Erosive leukoplakia requires prompt biopsy for early diagnosis of a possible malignancy.

Systemic

1. Pruritus can be controlled with antihistamines and mild sedatives.
2. In some patients, prolonged treatment with Etretinate (R.59) has shown good results in Europe and has recently been approved for use in the United States.

Topical

1. Testosterone propionate 2% in a fatty ointment can be used.
2. Regular skin care will prevent fissures and rhagades (R.31b).
3. Sitzbaths with tar or ichthyol additives, or both, and application of dye solutions (e.g., aqueous gentian violet solution [R.14a]) are indicated when marked irritation is present.
4. In some patients, short-term anti-inflammatory treatment with topical corticosteroids may be helpful. In women, this can be combined with estrogens.
5. In persistent cases, intralesional injections of corticosteroid crystal suspension may be indicated. The injections are very painful and may require general anesthesia.

Phimosis

Phimosis is a constriction of the foreskin present in newborn infants as a physiologic condition. Acquired phimoses are found as sequelae of balanitis xerotica obliterans (p. 165) and in balanoposthitis. Acute acquired phimoses occur in inflammatory diseases such as syphilis and genital herpes or with condylomata acuminata.

Paraphimosis is an acute complication of phimosis. If the phimotic prepuce becomes retracted, it can constrict the sulcus coronarius and cause massive edema of the distally located part of the prepuce (appearance of a Spanish collar). This constriction strangulates the blood supply and may result in gangrene of the glans unless reduction is accomplished within a few hours. This is best done in a very warm full bath after intravenous administration of an analgesic. If this is unsuccessful, surgical reduction by splitting the foreskin must be done as an emergency procedure followed by circumcision.

Severe congenital phimosis requires early circumcision as a prophylactic measure against balanitis and carcinoma of the penis.

Heterotopic Sebaceous Glands

Sebaceous glands can occasionally occur in increased numbers as yellowish pinhead-sized nodules on penis and prepuce and disquiet the patient. This is a variant of normal and is not a pathologic condition.

Hirsuties Papillaris Penis (Pearly Penile Papules)

These are embryologic remnants of a prehensile organ that develop after puberty and are present in approximately 10 per cent of the male population.

A seam of fine papillary proliferations can be seen at the junction of the glans penis with the sulcus coronarius. This is a variant of normal and does not require treatment.

Part III

Benign Tumors

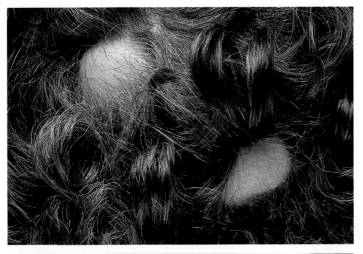

Figure 329. Atheromas (wen, pilar cyst): frequently seen on the scalp.

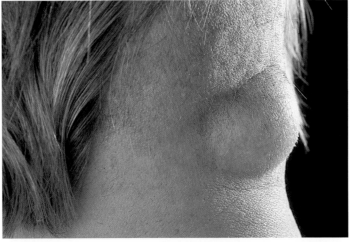

Figure 330. Atheroma of the neck (wen, pilar cyst).

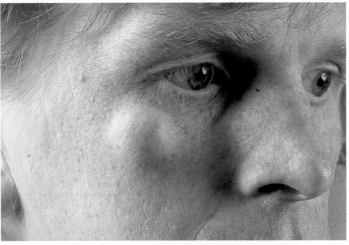

Figure 331. Retention cyst. Spheric, easily movable, firm tumor under tense but otherwise normal skin.

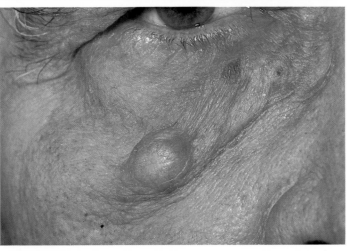

Figure 332. Retention cyst. Firm, well-demarcated tumor. Xanthelasma as an additional finding.

Atheromas, Retention Cysts

An atheroma (wen) is a cyst that occurs mainly on the scalp and originates from the epithelium of the hair follicle. It is also known as a trichilemmal cyst. These lesions show an autosomally dominant inheritance and occur as solitary lesions in approximately 30 per cent of all patients. In most patients, they occur as multiple lesions. Retention cysts (epidermoid cysts) occur more frequently and are difficult to distinguish from trichilemmal cysts. They originate from the ostium of the follicle and occur predominantly in men.

Clinical Appearance

Atheroma (Trichilemmal Cyst, Pilar Cyst)

1. Globular tense-elastic tumor, reaching the size of a plum, is freely movable on the underlying skin and is covered with atrophic, thin skin. The cysts have a thick wall and are filled with a white, pasty, keratinous material produced by the epithelium of the hair follicle. It is often easier to palpate than to visualize these lesions. There is no opening to the outside, as is often found in epidermoid cysts.
2. Atheromas (pilar cysts) are found almost exclusively on the scalp. On the larger cysts, the overlying skin is usually bald.
3. Trauma rarely causes inflammation or proliferation of the lesion. Malignant degeneration is almost never seen.

Retention Cysts (Epidermoid Cysts)

1. These are cutaneous or subcutaneous tumors of pinhead to plum size, depending on their developmental stage.
2. Areas of predilection are the face and trunk, but they can occur in all areas where hair follicles are present.
3. The cysts are ruptured easily with manipulation: the keratinous material escapes into the surrounding tissue, where it acts as a foreign body and causes the development of a granuloma. Secondary bacterial infection can produce abscess formation.
4. The expanded gland duct is frequently open, and the foul-smelling contents (rancid lipids and debris) can be evacuated. The cysts fill again after some time because the cyst wall remains intact.

Therapy

Repeated inflammation, proliferation, and other complications are indications for operative removal. An inflammation must be allowed to subside before surgery is performed. The cyst is removed by blunt enucleation with an attached spindle-shaped piece of skin. It is important to not leave remnants of the cyst, because a recurrence of the cyst can originate from these remnants. Scars from prior inflammations can make enucleation of the cyst technically difficult.

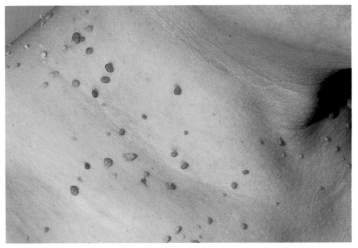

Figure 333. Pendulous fibromas (acrochordons). Soft, pedunculated, often pigmented tumors of the neck.

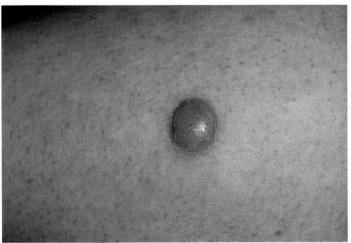

Figure 334. Histiocytoma (dermatofibroma). Lentil-sized, firm, slightly pigmented tumor.

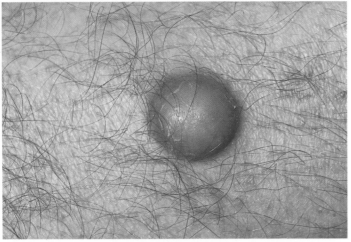

Figure 335. Histiocytoma (dermatofibroma). Typical appearance of the hemispheric, firm tumor with brownish margin (hemosiderin storage).

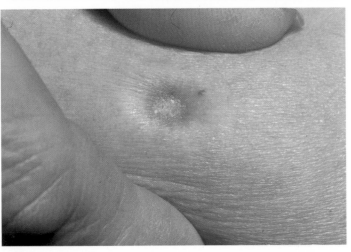

Figure 336. Histiocytoma (dermatofibroma). Firm tumor deeply embedded in the skin with depression of the overlying layers of the skin following tangential pressure.

Fibromas

Fibromas are frequently occurring benign neoplasms. They can be classified as soft pedunculated fibromas (fibroma molle, fibroma pendulans) and hard fibromas, such as histiocytomas or dermatofibromas. Histiocytomas occur mainly in young adults, especially on the extremities, and persist during the patient's entire lifetime without ever causing any symptoms. Malignant degeneration has not been reported in histiocytomas.

Fibroma Molle (Skin Tags)

Clinical Appearance

1. Soft fibromas are usually small, lentil- to pea-sized, pedunculated, skin-colored tumors. In rare cases, they can grow to the size of a small orange.
2. Fibroma pendulans is often found on the lateral aspects of the neck, on the shoulders, in the axillary and submammary regions, and occasionally in the inguinal area.
3. They often occur as multiple lesions. Obesity and hyperhidrosis predispose to the development of pedunculated fibromas.
4. Fibromas are mainly found in adults and can show a familial occurrence.
5. Soft fibromas occasionally become inflamed or show hemorrhagic infarction after torsion of the pedicle.

Therapy

Surgical removal is possible by electrocautery sling or scissors. The removal of large fibromas may be accompanied by considerable bleeding and require several sutures for wound closure.

Histiocytoma, Dermatofibroma

Clinical Appearance

1. These are hard, singular or multiple, hemispherical or disc-shaped nodules that are easily movable and rarely grow to more than 2 to 3 cm in size. Their color can be reddish or correspond to the color of the surrounding skin. Frequently, one sees a brownish discoloration from deposition of hemosiderin. Histiocytomas are usually raised above the level of the skin, but occasionally they can be slightly depressed and can then be palpated under the skin as hard nodules.
2. The areas of predilection are the extremities; the legs are affected more often than the arms.

Therapy

Treatment of these slow-growing tumors is usually not necessary as long as the diagnosis is confirmed. Tumors that cause cosmetic or diagnostic difficulties should be excised.

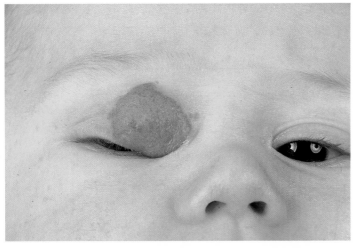

Figure 337. Capillary hemangioma of the upper eyelid.

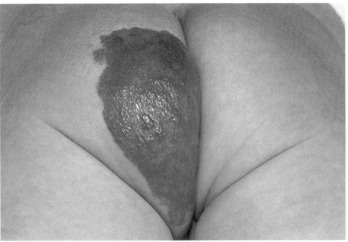

Figure 338. Capillary hemangioma in the gluteal area. Strawberry-like color and surface.

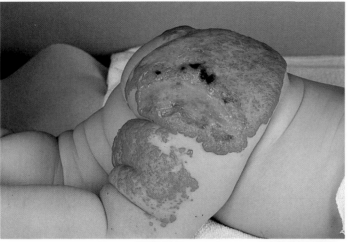

Figure 339. Capillary hemangioma. Ulceration and grayish discoloration as signs of beginning involution.

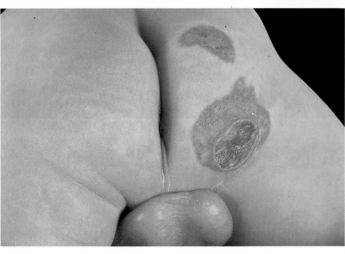

Figure 340. Capillary hemangiomas. Advanced involution with grayish discoloration and decrease of the tumors.

Hemangiomas

Vascular tumors are among the most frequent benign tumors of the skin. They can be distinguished on the basis of their clinical appearance and can be diagnosed without difficulty. Treatment usually depends on the type of tumor.

Capillary Hemangioma (Strawberry Nevus)

Capillary hemangioma occurs almost exclusively in children (in approximately 10 per cent of all children, two thirds girls, one third boys). It is rarely seen in adults. Practically all capillary hemangiomas involute spontaneously within a period of years, usually during childhood. The deep lesions involute later than the superficial ones do. Radical therapeutic measures should be avoided, if at all possible, since the tumors disappear spontaneously in almost all cases.

Clinical Appearance

1. This is a hemispherical or flat tumor that is bright red or bluish red in color. Occasionally, the tumors can show through the skin with a bluish color. Deep-seated lesions can be palpated as soft masses; the overlying skin may have normal color. The tumors occur as single or multiple lesions.
2. Larger hemangiomas can occasionally cause atrophy of the underlying bone.
3. Some capillary hemangiomas can ulcerate and are then covered with crusts. Serious bleeding from capillary hemangiomas is very rare.
4. These tumors can be located anywhere on the skin, including the face.
5. As the tumor involutes, its color gradually changes to gray. Eventually, only a flaccid sac remains that also involutes slowly.

Therapy

1. Treatment should be delayed as long as possible to await possible spontaneous involution of the lesion.
2. Operative treatment is indicated for tumors that impair breathing, eating, or other vital functions.
3. Other modes of treatment include radiation therapy and intralesional or systemic corticosteroids. These measures are indicated only in exceptional cases.

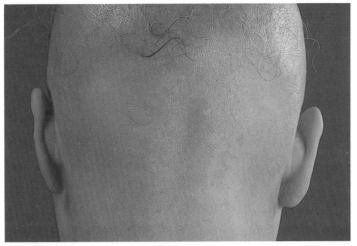

Figure 341. Median nevus flammeus of the neck. So-called "storkbite."

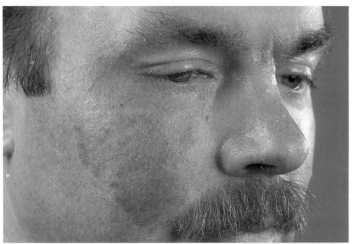

Figure 342. Lateral nevus flammeus in the distribution of the second trigeminus branch on the right.

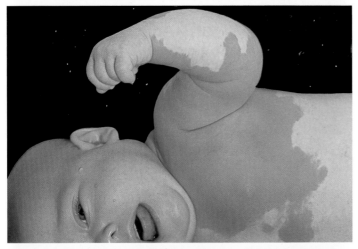

Figure 343. Hemilateral nevus flammeus.

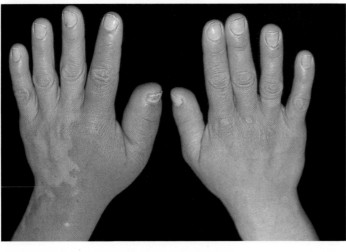

Figure 344. Nevus flammeus. Hypertrophy of thumb and index finger are clearly visible.

Nevus Flammeus, Port Wine Stain

Two clinical forms can be distinguished.

Median Nevus Flammeus

Discrete median or symmetric nevus flammeus is present at birth in two thirds of all children; the lesions disappear within the first year with a few exceptions (Unna-Pollitzer nevus nuchae, "stork bite").

Clinical Appearance

1. These are pale pink lesions in which telangiectasias are often clearly visible. The involved area is not elevated.
2. The lesions are always found in a median or symmetric location, especially on the neck, the midforehead, the glabellar region, and the eyelids.

Therapy

The lesion either disappears or regresses significantly during the first year of life. Treatment is not necessary.

Lateral Nevus Flammeus

This is the more striking form of nevus flammeus. It is present at birth and persists during the patient's entire life.

Clinical Appearance

1. The laterally located purple or deep red lesions can be only a few millimeters in size or cover a large area of skin. The surface is usually smooth.
2. These nevi flammei are usually unilateral. They can be irregular or show a segmental arrangement and are seen most often on the face and upper trunk.
3. The oral mucosa can be affected, especially with segmental involvement of the second and third branches of the trigeminal nerve.
4. In middle-aged or older patients, nevus flammeus can undergo cavernous changes. The cavernous segments of the tumor then become prominent.
5. Lateral nevi flammei can be associated with other developmental anomalies: Sturge-Weber syndrome (nevus flammeus in one or two adjacent segments of the trigeminal nerve, occasionally associated with glaucoma, amaurosis, convulsions, oligophrenia, and mental disorders); Klippel-Trenaunay syndrome (nevus flammeus, usually involving an entire extremity with bone and soft tissue hypertrophy and varicosities); or von Hippel-Lindau syndrome (nevus flammeus with cerebral, ocular, and many other symptoms).

Therapy

Treatment of these conditions is disappointing. In many cases, however, no treatment is necessary.
1. Conspicuous lesions can be hidden with water-insoluble makeup in the color of the surrounding skin.
2. Argon laser treatment can occasionally produce satisfactory cosmetic results.
3. Attempts to obliterate the enlarged blood vessels with diathermy or by injection of sclerosing solutions have shown disappointing cosmetic results.

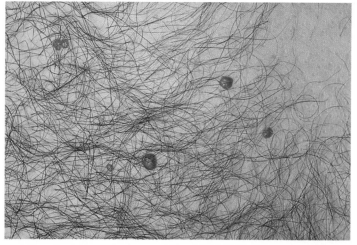

Figure 345. Senile angiomas (cherry angiomas). Medium to dark red approximately lentil-sized tumors. Normal finding of senile skin.

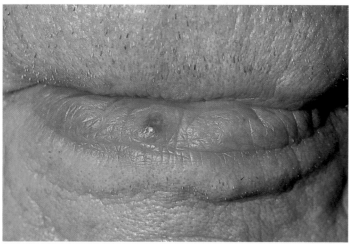

Figure 346. Senile angioma in the red of the lip that is of blue-red to dark blue color in this location.

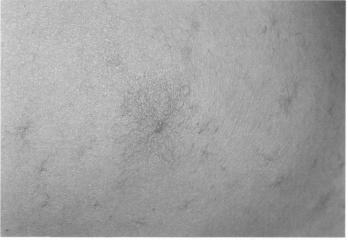

Figure 347. Spider telangiectases. Central, occasionally pulsating prominence with stellate-shaped efferent blood vessel dilatations.

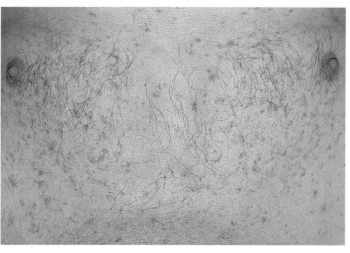

Figure 348. Multiple spider telangiectases in a patient with cirrhosis of the liver.

Senile Angiomas

These are benign tumors (aggregates of enlarged blood vessels). They are a normal finding in the skin of elderly people.

Clinical Appearance
1. Pinhead to pea-sized light to dark red tumors that never bleed are characteristic.
2. They are found primarily on the trunk, the extremities, and the face.

Therapy
No treatment is necessary.

Spider Telangiectasia (Nevus Araneus)

Spider telangiectasias may be nevoid (nevus araneus) or acquired. They are seen in healthy people, in patients with chronic liver disease, with estrogen therapy, and during pregnancy.

Clinical Appearance
1. A pulsating central arteriole (loupe, pressure with glass spatula) with stellate efferent blood-filled capillaries is typical for this lesion.
2. Spider telangiectasias are located mainly on the face, the chest, and the upper back, less often on the back of the neck or the dorsum of the hand.
3. A palmar erythema can be an associated symptom, with or without liver disease.
4. In patients with cirrhosis of the liver, spider telangiectasias can occasionally grow to penny-sized lesions with a prominent central arteriole. Abrupt arterial bleeding either spontaneously or with minimal trauma can, rarely, occur with these lesions.

Therapy
Spider telangiectasias that develop during pregnancy involute spontaneously. Most other spider telangiectasias can involute partially; most of these lesions persist, however.

Therapy may be indicated for cosmetic reasons. Electrocautery with a diathermy needle is an effective method; the central arteriole must be obliterated. If unsuccessful, cautery can be repeated after several weeks. Local anesthesia is not always necessary.

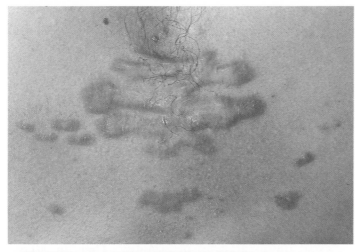

Figure 349. Keloids. So-called spontaneous keloids in the center of the chest as a sequel of acne vulgaris.

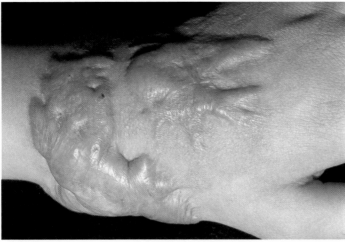

Figure 350. Burn keloids.

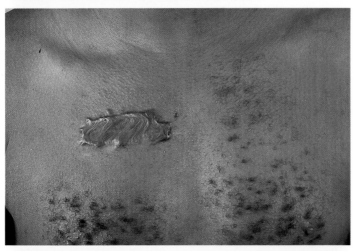

Figure 351. Pigmented keloid in a black patient. Racial disposition. Partial involution after treatment with a pressure pad.

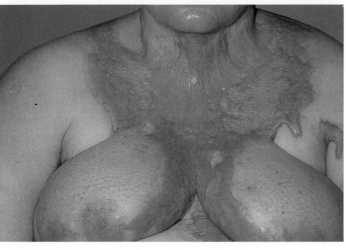

Figure 352. Extensive keloid formation in burn scars. There is also distinct scar contracture in the neck area.

Keloids

Keloids are circumscribed formations of hypertrophied fibrous tissue. They usually occur after injuries, especially after thermal and chemical burns. Spontaneous keloids can develop without preceding trauma. There appears to be a genetic disposition for keloid formation; keloids are known to show a familial tendency. They occur more frequently in blacks and Asians. Certain skin diseases, especially acne, also represent a predisposition for keloids. Hypertrophic scars must be distinguished from keloids, even though they have a similar appearance clinically and histologically. They develop without a special disposition after injuries or in operative scars that do not correspond to relaxed skin tension lines.

Clinical Appearance

1. Keloids are sharply delineated firm fibrous tissue excrescences of reddish color that can develop at the site of a preceding injury or may occur spontaneously. Telangiectatic, enlarged blood vessels are visible occasionally. The overlying skin is often atrophic and thin without follicle openings or hairs.
2. Keloids are found most often on the upper body, especially on the face, the neck, and the upper part of the trunk, especially in the presternal region.
3. The lesions are tender, hyperaesthetic, and pruritic.

Therapy

An effective systemic therapy for keloids does not exist.

1. Regression of fresh keloids can be achieved with topical corticosteroid treatment under an occlusive foil (R.36), or better with intralesional injections of corticosteroid crystal suspension (R.44).
2. Circumscribed firm keloid strands can be softened by frequent massages with bland ointments.
3. A pressure pad worn like a truss can, in some cases, cause a certain regression of the keloid.
4. Surgical procedures should be used only in selected cases; a new keloid often forms after excision. One can try to suppress this renewed keloid formation by immediate injection of a corticosteroid crystal suspension (or with radiation therapy). Excision of hypertrophic scars with revision of the incision (Z-plasty, and so on) often produces a satisfactory cosmetic result.

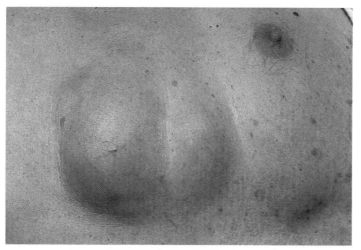

Figure 353. Lipoma. Soft, subcutaneus tumor with septum formation.

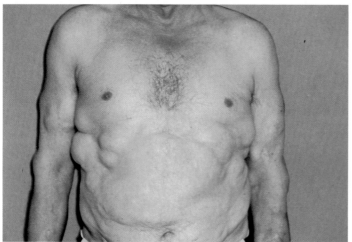

Figure 354. Benign symmetric lipomatosis. Multiple lipomas with a largely symmetric arrangement.

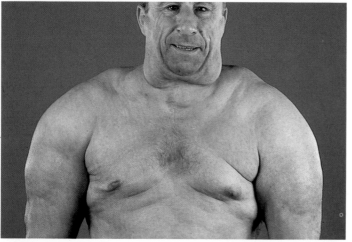

Figure 355. Benign symmetric lipomatosis with a so-called Madelung's fat neck. Multiple widespread symmetric lipomas simulate an athletic habitus.

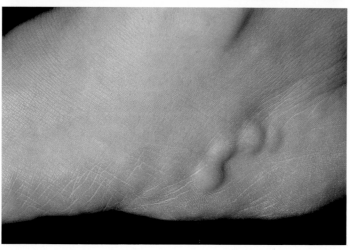

Figure 356. Painful piezogenic pedal papules (PPPP). Small, occasionally painful, fat hernias on the heel.

Lipomas, Lipomatosis

Lipomas are seen as solitary or multiple lipomas, usually without other symptoms. They can also occur as part of other diseases, especially benign symmetric lipomatosis, occasionally in Gardner syndrome, and in neurofibromatosis (von Recklinghausen's disease).

Solitary or Multiple Lipomas

Lipomas are benign tumors of fatty tissue that can occur as solitary or multiple lesions (multiple in 7 per cent of all lipoma patients). Multiple lipomas can appear as a few or multiple lesions in an irregular, asymmetric distribution. They can be diffuse or limited to certain regions without showing a defined syndrome into which a particular lipomatosis can be classified. These multiple lipomas and solitary lipomas have no sexual preference. The cause of the disorder is not known.

Clinical Appearance

1. This is a slowly developing, soft, smooth, flat tumor.
2. These tumors can be found in any region of the body that contains fatty tissue, including the oral mucosa. Lipomas are seen most frequently in areas containing much subcutaneous fat, especially the trunk and the extremities. Solitary and multiple lipomas occur in an irregular and disseminated fashion, in contrast to benign symmetric lipomatosis.
3. Any lipoma can be painful during a growth spurt, especially individual or numerous lipomas of a lipomatosis. Solitary lipomas are rarely painful.

Therapy

No therapy is necessary when the diagnosis is confirmed. Surgical treatment may be necessary for cosmetic reasons or when the tumor causes excessive pressure.

Benign Symmetric Lipomatosis (Madelung Syndrome)

Multiple lipomas are the leading symptom of benign symmetric lipomatosis, a rare, nonhereditary disease that affects men five times more often than it does women. The disease usually occurs between the thirtieth and fiftieth year of life.

Clinical Appearance

1. Multiple soft or firm symmetrically arranged lipomas with a typical distribution are characteristic.
2. Lipomas are located most often in the neck or posterior neck region, presenting the clinical appearance of a Fetthals of Madelung or a buffalo neck. Other lipomas are frequently found on the head, the upper trunk, and the proximal parts of the upper extremities.
3. Lipomas can remain unchanged for many years and then grow rapidly for some time. During these periods of rapid growth, they can be painful, either spontaneously or upon pressure. In rare instances, lipomas can develop in the respiratory, the gastrointestinal, and the urogenital tracts, very rarely in other organs.
4. Some of these patients have pathologic changes of the liver from alcohol abuse. Hyperuricemia and rheumatoid joint pains can also exist.

Therapy

Causal therapy can only be directed against an underlying disease. In most cases, no treatment is possible. Impairment of vital functions (e.g., narrowing of respiratory pathways) may be an indication for surgical removal of the lipomas.

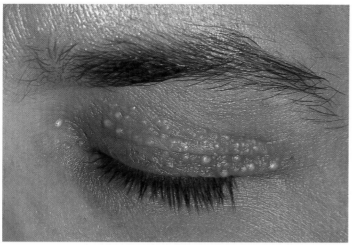

Figure 357. Milia of the upper eyelid. Whitish, reactionless keratin cysts.

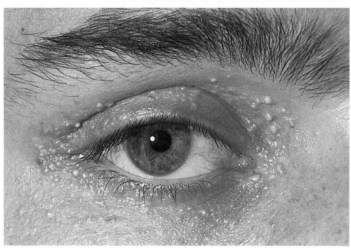

Figure 358. Milia. Extensive involvement around the eye.

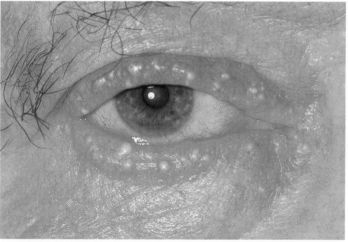

Figure 359. Extensive milia involvement in a patient with mycosis fungoides.

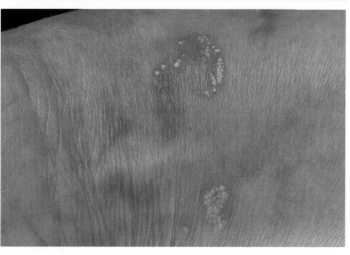

Figure 360. So-called post-inflammatory milia, usually as a sequel of subepidermal bullae (in this patient secondary to bullous pemphigoid).

Milia

Milia are small subepidermal keratinous cysts. They occur from childhood to old age and are mainly of cosmetic significance. Occasionally, milia are the result of excessive exposure to sunlight. Multiple milia can develop rapidly, in an eruptive manner, especially in young women. They can also be the result of subepidermal blister formation, e.g., after burns, porphyria cutanea tarda, bullous pemphigoid, or epidermolysis bullosa. Occasionally, they are found in patients with mycosis fungoides and cortisone-induced atrophy of the skin and after radiation therapy.

Clinical Appearance

1. White or yellow flat tumors, 1 to 2 mm in diameter are characteristic.
2. They usually are located in the face, especially around the eyes, on the eyelids, and on the cheeks.

Therapy

Incision of the epidermis over the milium with needle or scalpel and subsequent expression of the cyst is a simple and effective treatment.

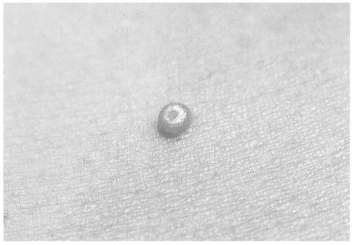

Figure 361. Molluscum contagiosum. Glassy, pitted nodule.

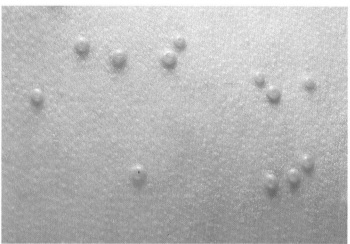

Figure 362. Mollusca contagiosa. Dissemination of glassy, in some cases pitted, nodules without inflammatory reaction.

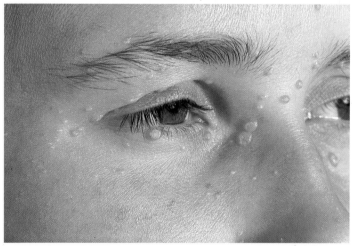

Figure 363. Mollusca contagiosa. Dense involvement with mostly pitted, round tumors of varying sizes.

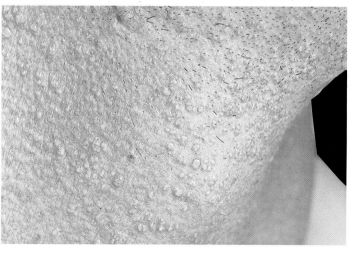

Figure 364. Mollusca contagiosa. Exanthematous dissemination on skin that had been treated with cortisone.

Molluscum Contagiosum

Mollusca contagiosa are seen most frequently in children but are also seen very often in adults. They are a form of warts, caused by a virus, and are spread by infection. In contrast to other infectious warts, they are not caused by papilloma virus but by a pox virus. Children with atopic dermatitis and patients with immunodeficiency from corticosteroid and cytostatic therapy are especially susceptible. In most cases, these patients are otherwise healthy. Mollusca contagiosa usually heal approximately 6 months to 3 years after the eruptions begin. The infection is transmitted by direct contact; in adults, it can be transmitted by sexual intercourse. The time of incubation is 2 to 3 weeks. The disease often spreads by autoinoculation.

Clinical Appearance

1. Skin-colored to pearl white, waxy, dome-shaped or umbilicated tumors 2 to 10 mm in size appear in large numbers or at least as multiple lesions. The pitted tumors are distributed on the skin in an asymmetric fashion, often in groups or disseminated. They do not show increased keratinization like verrucae vulgares.
2. The neck and trunk, especially the axillary and genital regions, are areas of predilection, but the lips, tongue, and oral mucosa can also be affected.
3. Inflammatory erythema, pustules, and crusts can develop spontaneously or after scratching, especially where solitary or only a few mollusca contagiosa are present. This can make the diagnosis difficult in some cases; the lesions are otherwise easy to diagnose (typical appearance, multiple lesions).

Therapy

The disease is harmless and usually heals spontaneously; only those treatment methods that do not result in scars should be employed.

1. When only a few mollusca are present, they can be removed with a curette under local anesthesia (freezing with ethyl chloride).
2. Incision of the epidermis overlying the molluscum and expression of the whitish contents is another successful treatment method.
3. For widespread involvement, Vitamin A treatment can be tried, for sensitive skin as an ointment (R.42b), in all other cases as a gel (R.24b) or solution.
4. In cases with widespread involvement, especially in children, the patients may have to be hospitalized for removal of the mollusca under general anesthesia.

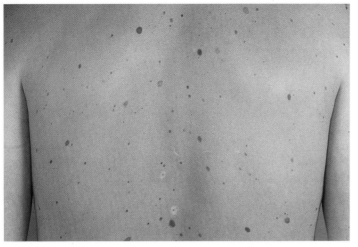

Figure 365. Nevus-cell nevus. Normal spectrum of pigmented nevi.

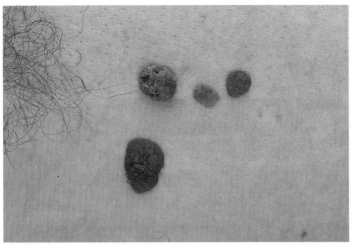

Figure 366. Nevus-cell nevi. Mulberry-shaped, exophytic growing pigmented nevi.

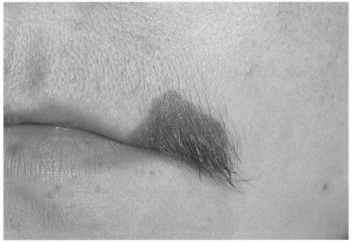

Figure 367. Nevus-cell nevi. Nevus pigmentosus et pilosus with increased hair growth. This occurs frequently in large nevus-cell nevi.

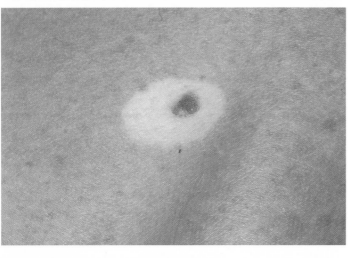

Figure 368. Sutton nevus. Nevus-cell nevus with sharply demarcated, depigmented halo.

Pigmented Nevi

Nevus-Cell Nevus

Nevus-cell nevi are benign tumors of normal skin that develop through proliferation of nevocytes. They can be found in practically all people. At birth, only a few individual nevus-cell nevi are present; they increase in number in the first years of life and reach a maximum of 30 to 50 nevus-cell nevi in the third and fourth decade. After that, they gradually decrease (partly with pigment loss and fibrous tissue formation). A few isolated nevus-cell nevi can develop in old age. Nevus-cell nevi must be distinguished from malignant melanoma. Rapid growth, change in color, or weeping, bleeding, and pruritus should make one suspect a malignancy. Early stages of malignant melanoma (see p. 215) are difficult to distinguish from nevus-cell nevus. A dermatologist experienced in dermatologic oncology should be consulted.

Clinical Appearance

1. Nevus-cell nevi develop very slowly. Almost all stages of development are usually present, from light or dark brown, very flat, round tumors of 1 to 2 mm to a soft more prominent tumor in all shades of brown. Nevus-cell nevi are often hairy, with thick brown hair.
2. They are usually distributed over the entire skin in an irregular fashion.
3. Nevus-cell nevi do not occur on the oral mucosa. Nevi on the red of the lips are usually nevi spili and not nevus-cell nevi.

Therapy

With the exception of giant hairy nevi (see further on), nevus-cell nevi do not require treatment other than an occasional diagnostic biopsy. Offensive nevus-cell nevi may occasionally have to be removed for cosmetic reasons. Incomplete removal or trauma to a nevus-cell nevus does not carry the risk of malignant degeneration.

Sutton's Nevus, Halo Nevus

This is a special form of nevus-cell nevus characterized by a round, depigmented halo surrounding a pigmented or nonpigmented nevus-cell nevus. Later, the central nevus-cell nevus can disappear, and only the round leukodermic area remains. Eventually this, too, can disappear through repigmentation. Sutton's nevi can develop as solitary or multiple lesions in between other less conspicuous nevus-cell nevi and alarm the patient. They are not malignant and excision is not absolutely necessary.

Giant Hairy Nevus

Giant hairy nevi are large, usually hairy, nevus-cell nevi that are present at birth, occasionally as multiple lesions. They do not disappear spontaneously. Depending on their distribution, they may be known as bathing trunk nevi, and so on. Malignant degeneration of a giant hairy nevus occurs somewhat more frequently than it does in nevus-cell nevi. Histologically, the appearance of a giant hairy nevus can be similar to that of a malignant melanoma, for which it is sometimes mistaken.

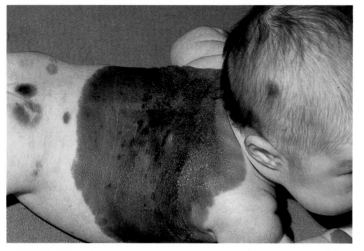

Figure 369. Nevus giganteus. Multiple, congenital nevus-cell nevi with varying pigmentation.

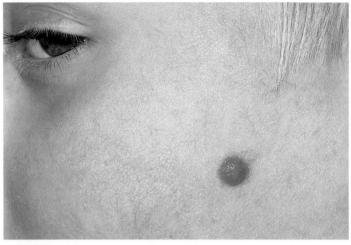

Figure 370. Spitz nevus (juvenile melanoma). Reddened hemispheric tumor with smooth surface.

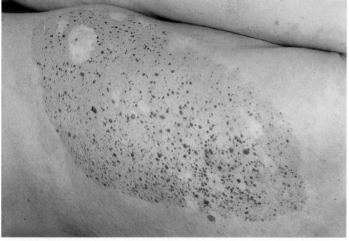

Figure 371. Nevus spilus. Widespread sharply demarcated light brown discoloration with multiple enclosed nevus-cell nevi.

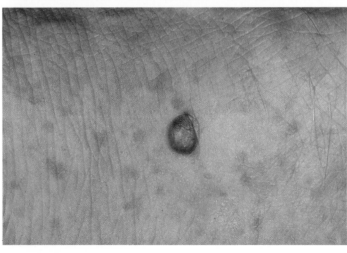

Figure 372. Blue nevus. Firm, blue-black tumor.

<table>
<tr><td>Clinical Appearance</td><td>Involvement of the nervous system is possible in rare cases.</td></tr>
</table>

Clinical Appearance

Involvement of the nervous system is possible in rare cases.

1. The often large tumor is usually dark brown, but segments of it can occasionally be a lighter brown. Its surface is smooth or a papillomatous soft. The tumor is often covered with thick brown-black hair that can form vertices.
2. The size of the tumors can vary considerably; they can be coin-size tumors or may cover large areas of the body, for instance, an entire extremity.
3. All parts of the body can be involved.

Therapy

1. Surgical removal of an unsuspicious giant hairy nevus may be indicated if the patient desires it. It is often necessary for cosmetic reasons, but complete removal may require several stages with subsequent plastic procedures for coverage. Large tumors cannot always be removed completely.
2. Dermabrasion is useful only in infants. The patient must be hospitalized, and the operation is performed under general anesthesia.

Spitz Nevus (Juvenile Melanoma)

This always benign, often pigment-poor, tumor occurs mainly in children and only rarely in adults. It is a special form of a pigment cell nevus that may resemble a malignant melanoma histologically.

Clinical Appearance

1. A round, hemispheric, or cone-shaped tumor usually develops in early childhood. It is well vascularized and, therefore, red, reddish-brown, or (rarely) brown in color. These tumors grow to a maximal size of 1 to 2 cm in diameter. The surface is sometimes fragile and crusty; minimal trauma can cause bleeding.
2. The most frequent location is the face, especially the cheeks, followed by the legs and other areas of the skin.

Therapy

Treatment of choice is surgical excision of the tumor in order to confirm the diagnosis histologically; conservative excision is sufficient.

Nevus Spilus

Clinical Appearance

Nevi spili are sharply delineated, light brown discolorations that may or may not be speckled with lentigines or nevus-cell nevi. They occur frequently as harmless solitary lesions. Multiple nevi spili are found as café au lait spots in neurofibromatosis von Recklinghausen.

Therapy

Removal of nevi spili is not necessary.

Blue Nevus

These are very slowly growing blue or blue-black tumors consisting of pigmented melanocytes. They are located deep in the dermis, which causes their blue color. Blue nevi can be present at birth or can develop later in life. Malignant degeneration appears to be extremely rare and has been reported in only a few isolated cases.

Clinical Appearance

1. The tumors are usually flat, occasionally raised in a nodular fashion; their surface is smooth. They are dark blue, sometimes with a gray to whitish center, and are rarely more than 1 cm in diameter.
2. Blue nevi are found mainly on the extremities, especially on the back of the hands, the feet, the buttocks, and the face.

Therapy

Operative removal is not necessary as long as one is sure of the diagnosis. Excisional biopsy should include the subcutaneous tissue, because blue nevi are often located deep in the dermis.

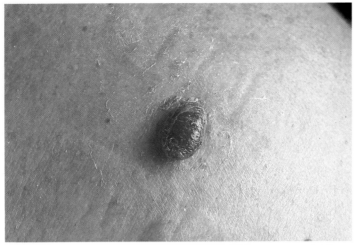

Figure 373. Pyogenic granuloma. Intensively reddened, soft tumor with surrounding raised and scaling margin. The surface is very friable.

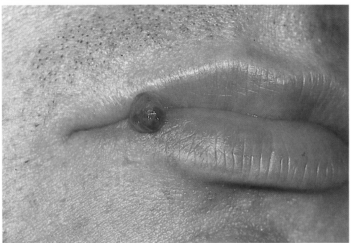

Figure 374. Pyogenic granuloma. Easily bleeding, erosive, pedunculated tumor on the lower lip.

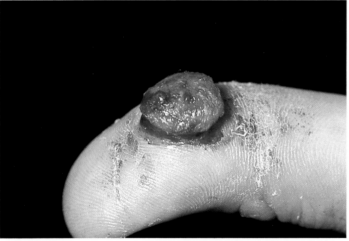

Figure 375. Pyogenic granuloma. Superficially eroded tumor with small base that developed rapidly after an injury.

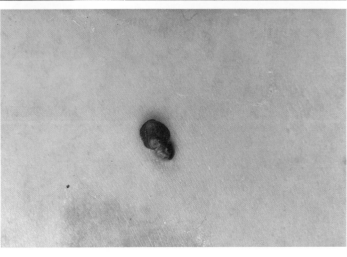

Figure 376. Pyogenic granuloma. Black tumor caused by hemorrhagic infarction. The tumor simulates a malignant melanoma.

Pyogenic Granuloma

Granuloma Telangiectaticum

These are tumor-like growths of fresh, well-vascularized granulation tissue that develop a few weeks after minor injuries. They are not infectious. Since they grow rapidly, weep, and bleed easily, these tumors are often mistaken for malignant lesions, especially malignant melanomas. Pyogenic granulomas occasionally show a tendency for recurrent bleeding. They occur frequently in children, in young adults, and during pregnancy. The diagnosis is based on the rapid growth and the clinical appearance of a well-vascularized and friable tumor. Histologic examination is absolutely necessary, because the clinical diagnosis is often misleading. Differential diagnoses include seborrheic warts with inflammatory changes, nevus-cell nevi, mollusca contagiosa, and angiomas.

Clinical Appearance

1. Pyogenic granulomas are red, occasionally red-brown or blue-black, soft, nontender tumors that can be sessile with a broad base or, more rarely, pedunculated. They measure 5 to 10 mm in diameter and are surrounded by an epithelial wreath. Their surface can be smooth or erosive, occasionally weeping or bleeding, or covered by a yellowish layer of fibrin. Spontaneous involution occurs rarely when the hemorrhagic black tumor dries up.
2. Most frequent locations are the hands, especially the fingers, the feet (toes), lips, head, and trunk.
3. The oral mucosa, especially the gingiva, can also be involved (epulis telangiectatica, epulis of pregnancy).

Therapy

1. The treatment of choice is complete excision; remnants often lead to a recurrence. The excised tissue should always be examined histologically.
2. The tumor can also be removed with a curette or by electrocoagulation.

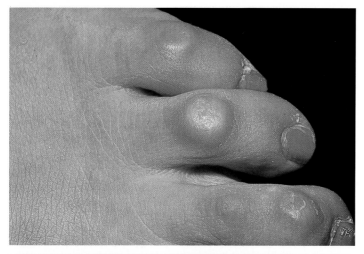

Figure 377. Clavi, corns. Round, painful callosities of the toes.

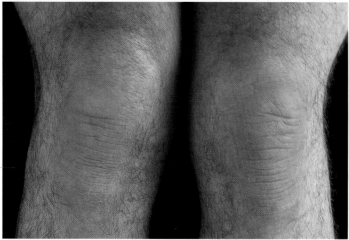

Figure 378. Floor-layer's knee. Chronic inflammation and thickening of the skin from prolonged kneeling.

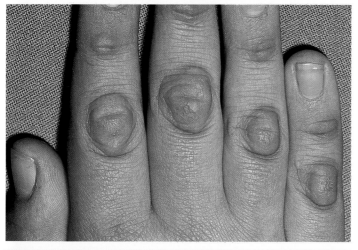

Figure 379. Knuckle pads. Circumscribed, callus-like thickening of the skin over the finger joints.

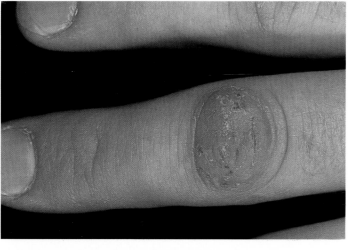

Figure 380. Callus caused by chewing. Circumscribed inflammation and reactive callus formation caused by habitual chewing on the knuckle.

Callosities

These circumscribed hyperkeratoses are reactions of the skin to chronic intermittent mechanical irritations. The tendency to form callosities varies significantly among individuals. Location of the callus is often an indication of a special activity or occupation, but callosities can also be stigmata of bad habits (chewing, sucking). Callus formation is a protective mechanism of the skin, and only rarely the symptom of a disease.

Clinical Appearance

1. Circumscribed hyperkeratosis in the area of increased pressure is characteristic.
2. Callosities form mainly on the palms of the hands and soles of the feet. They may develop in other locations as stigmata of certain occupations (milker's callus, floor layer's knee, or trumpeter's lip).
3. Callosities are not tender. They disappear completely after cessation of the pressure.
4. A clavus (corn) is a special type of callosity that can be extremely painful. Clavi develop as round hyperkeratoses with central cores over bony prominences of the feet from pressure or friction, especially when improper shoes are worn or abnormalities of the foot skeleton are present. Irritation of the underlying dermis causes inflammation and irritation of sensory nerves resulting in marked tenderness.

Therapy

Ordinarily, callosities do not require treatment; within the limits of normal, they are a desirable protective reaction of the skin against increased mechanical pressure. Callosities that are the result of "bad habits" usually disappear when these activities are eliminated.

Therapy of clavi consists of softening the hyperkeratotic tissue with salicylic acid–containing plasters or a corresponding solution (salicylic acid solution, lactic acid solution). The hyperkeratotic tissue can then be removed easily, after a hot foot bath. After removal, the most important task is the prevention of a recurrent clavus. The patient must be advised to buy proper footwear and to relieve pressure on the areas exposed to mechanical stress by application of felt donuts or rings. Patients with foot deformities should be referred to an orthopedist for evaluation and correction of these problems. Procedures with scalpel or curette should be avoided in patients with diabetes or arterial occlusive disease. Even minor trauma can cause gangrene or malum perforans.

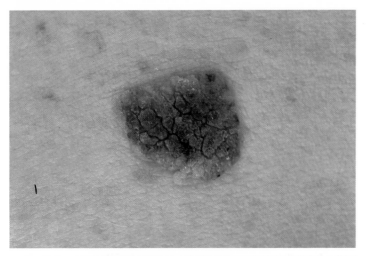

Figure 381. Seborrheic keratosis. Slightly raised tumor with fissured surface and fatty crumbly coating.

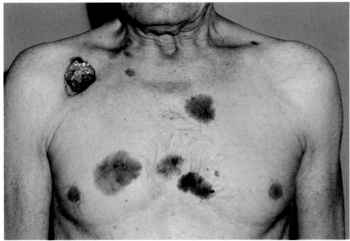

Figure 382. Seborrheic keratosis. Several unusually large tumors with varying pigmentation.

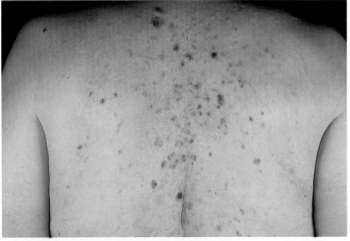

Figure 383. Multiple seborrheic keratoses on the patient's back.

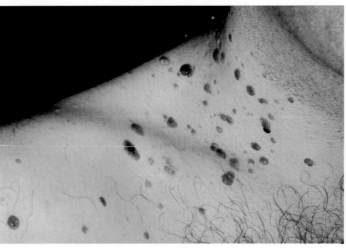

Figure 384. Multiple small seborrheic keratoses on the lateral aspect of the neck.

Seborrheic Keratosis

Seborrheic warts are seen very frequently. The patients are not greatly affected by them and often accept them as inevitable stigmata of aging. Men and women are affected equally. There is often a familial tendency. Typical seborrheic warts are rarely found before the fifth decade of life. Since pigmented spots are biopsied and examined histologically more often today, early stages of seborrheic warts are frequently diagnosed in the third or fourth decade.

In most cases, seborrheic warts are harmless symptoms of aging. Rarely, the sudden appearance of multiple seborrheic warts may be associated with a malignant tumor. Malignant degeneration of seborrheic warts has not been reported.

Clinical Appearance

1. Seborrheic warts are sharply demarcated, initially flat, lentil- to coin-size areas with brown pigmentation. With time, they develop into papillomatous, hemispherically raised tumors with light to dark brown pigmentation. They are soft, crumbly, and seborrheic. On close examination, one can distinguish horny cores in the follicle openings.
2. Seborrheic warts can develop in any area with sebaceous glands, most frequently on the trunk and in the face. They are not seen on the soles and the palms. Large, "granulated" seborrheic warts are seen mainly in the face and on the scalp.
3. Irritation can cause crust formation on the surface and inflammation at the base, which may make differentiation from squamous cell carcinoma or malignant melanoma difficult.

Therapy

Seborrheic warts are harmless, and their removal is usually not necessary. They should be removed if a malignant tumor cannot be excluded, such as basal cell epithelioma or malignant melanoma. Other indications for removal are frequent or severe irritation or are cosmetic. Other methods of removal, other than excision, are removal with a diathermy sling or a curette following electrocautery or freezing with ethyl chloride (caution: risk of explosion). These are tissue-destructive procedures and should be used only when the diagnosis is confirmed.

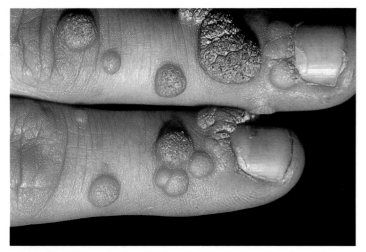

Figure 385. Verrucae vulgares. Tumors of varying keratinization, especially on the groove of the nail.

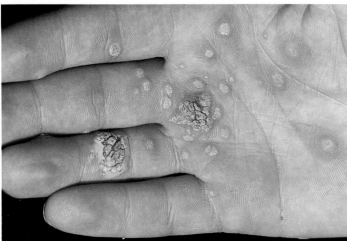

Figure 386. Multiple verrucae vulgares on the palm of the hand.

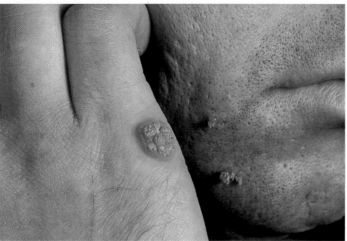

Figure 387. Filiform verrucae vulgares in the face, transmitted through contact with the hand.

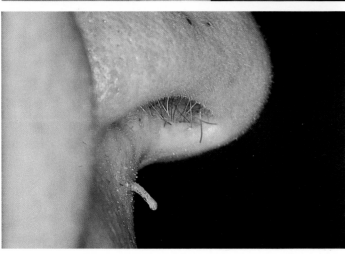

Figure 388. Filiform wart below the nose.

Warts

Infectious warts are papules induced on skin and mucous membranes by human papilloma virus. They can be classified according to clinical, histologic, and virologic criteria. For practical purposes, the clinical classification is most useful. It distinguishes between common warts (verrucae vulgares), plantar warts (verrucae plantares), flat warts (verrucae planae juveniles), epidermodysplasia verruciformis, and condylomata acuminata. The time of incubation is several weeks to several months. The clinical manifestations after contact with the infectious organism are determined by the patient's disposition. These predisposing factors include cool, moist acra and impairment of the immune system (atopic dermatitis, malignant tumors, cytostatic therapy, and so on). In immunodepressed patients, multiple common warts often occur in a disseminated fashion.

Common Warts (Verrucae Vulgares)

Clinical Appearance

1. Common warts are firm nodules with verrucous rough surfaces. They range in size from pinhead to pea size and can coalesce to form widespread beds of warts.
2. They are mainly located on the dorsum of hands and fingers but can occur in any other part of the body. Common warts occur chiefly in children.
3. Common warts usually disappear spontaneously in children, generally after 6 to 12 months, in adults after 12 to 24 months. They do not leave scars. Pressure from warts near the nailbed can cause permanent impairment of nail growth.

Therapy

Aggressive therapeutic measures should be avoided, since common warts heal without scars after a relatively limited period of time. A more intensive treatment may be indicated for widespread involvement of hands and feet and to prevent further dissemination of the warts. Therapeutic measures in use today are based on physical or chemical destruction of the warts.

1. Salicylic acid–containing plasters or other film-forming solutions are used to soften the hyperkeratotic material.
2. Two or three days later, the hyperkeratotic tissue is removed with a curette after a hot bath. The procedure may have to be repeated several times.
3. Freezing with liquid nitrogen is an alternative. The wart can then be removed together with the blister caused by the freezing. This method is very effective, but it is not very economical to keep a supply of liquid nitrogen in the physician's office. Cryotherapy is effective in 50 per cent of the patients but may be painful when used for treatment of periungual and plantar warts.
4. For chemical treatment, a cytostatic drug (5-fluorouracil) in DMSO is available in Europe. This drug must be applied to the affected areas regularly up to four times daily for several weeks. As long as the treated areas are small, there will be no systemic effect.
5. Contrast baths stimulate the blood flow.
6. Excision of the warts with a scalpel cannot be recommended. It results in scar formation and is plagued by frequent recurrences.
7. Radiation therapy of common warts is obsolete.
8. Biting and chewing promotes spreading of common warts (autoinoculation) and should be avoided.

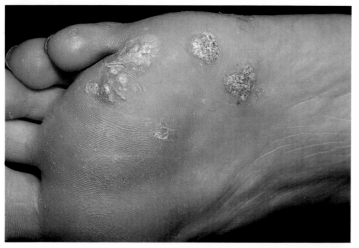

Figure 389. Plantar warts. Aggregated, very painful, keratotic tumors, which are not very exophytic due to the constant pressure.

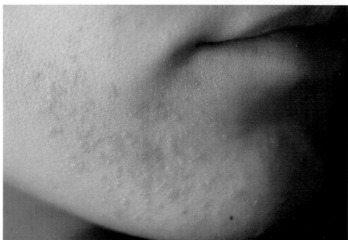

Figure 390. Verrucae planae juveniles. Slightly raised, skin-colored to slightly brown, often multiple tumors that are frequently located in the face, as in this case.

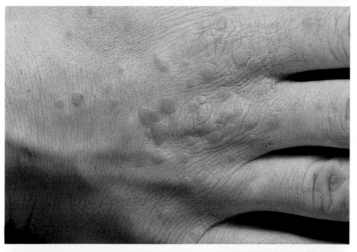

Figure 391. Verrucae planae juveniles. Multiple slightly raised, skin-colored to slightly reddened tumors.

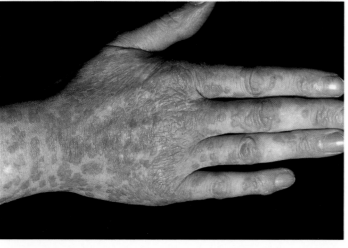

Figure 392. Epidermodysplasia verruciformis generalisata Lewandowsky-Lutz. Exanthematic dissemination of densely arranged flat warts.

Plantar Warts

Clinical Appearance

Warts on the soles of the feet have a distinctive appearance caused by the constant mechanical pressure. Multiple flat warts may be arranged in patches and are called mosaic warts; circumscribed solitary warts with cone-shaped extensions into the deep tissue are known as thorny warts. The constant pressure on the sole forces the corneous material into the deep tissues; the cone-shaped extension is usually covered by a callus. These lesions are very painful.

Therapy

1. Topical therapy is the same as that described for verrucae vulgares.
2. Pressure on the lesion should be relieved by application of felt rings and shoe inserts that allow the wart to grow outward. This also results in significant pain relief.
3. For persistent plantar warts that continue to recur at the same site, orthopedic consultation for possible skeletal deformities of the foot may be indicated.
4. Patients who are prone to develop plantar warts should avoid going barefoot in places where plantar warts are easily acquired, such as swimming pools and washrooms.
5. There should be no radiation therapy of the soles (or palms).

Flat Juvenile Warts (Verruca Plana Juvenilis)

Clinical Appearance

1. Soft flat or slightly raised, skin-colored to light yellow nodules are characteristic. They are often visible only with a loupe in oblique light.
2. Sites of predilection are the face (may be spread by shaving) and the dorsum of the hand.
3. These warts frequently develop primarily as multiple lesions. They can persist for a long time and respond poorly to therapeutic measures. They often disappear spontaneously after 6 to 24 months.

Therapy

1. In men, warts in appropriate locations can be hidden by a beard until they heal spontaneously.
2. Lesions that are not too extensive can be treated with topical applications of preparations containing lactic acid plus salicylic acid (Duofilm, Tiflex) or fluorouracil (Efudex, Fluoroplex).
3. The skin can be peeled with Vitamin A preparations (for sensitive skin as a cream [R.42b]) or as a gel [R.24b]). Therapy may have to be interrupted temporarily if the skin becomes too irritated.

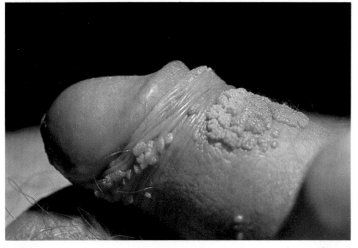

Figure 393. Condylomata acuminata. Soft skin colored to slightly whitish virus-papillomata in a grapelike aggregation.

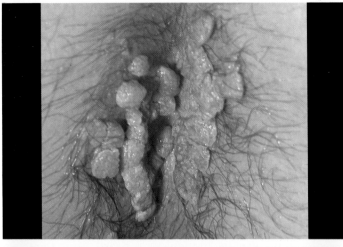

Figure 394. Condylomata acuminata. Perianal, weeping condyloma aggregation.

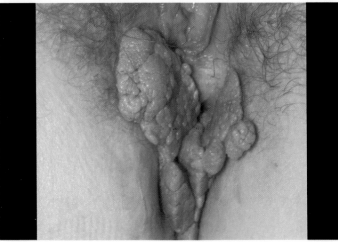

Figure 395. Condylomata acuminata. Extensive involvement of papillomatous tumors, partly flattened by compression.

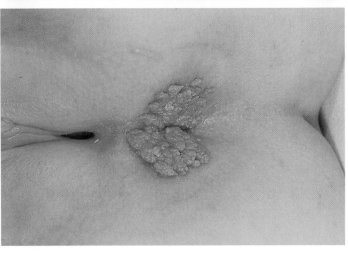

Figure 396. Perianal condylomata acuminata in a 5-year-old girl.

Epidermodysplasia Verruciformis

This is a rare disease with a genetic disposition in which multiple warts develop, especially in light-exposed areas of the body. The disease must be taken seriously because individual warts can develop into malignant tumors.

Condylomata Acuminata

These are a clinical variety of virus-induced warts that occur only in the anogenital area. They are sexually transmitted and have an incubation period of up to 8 months. Condylomata acuminata can disappear spontaneously within months or several years. Whenever condylomata acuminata are present, the diagnostic workup should always include other venereal diseases, such as AIDS, gonorrhea, syphilis, trichomoniasis, and chlamydial infections.

Clinical Appearance

1. The initial lesion is a pinhead-size pink to whitish nodule. As the disease progresses, a typical morphologic appearance develops with beds of warts and cauliflower-like masses that can eventually involve the entire anogenital region through autoinoculation.
2. In women, condylomata acuminata are found mostly on labia majora et minora but can be spread into the vagina and the cervix uteri. In men, the main locations are sulcus coronarius and the mucous membrane of the prepuce. Involvement of the urethra is also possible. Condylomata acuminata of the perianal region may involve the mucous membrane of the anus, and a recurrence often originates from these lesions.
3. The accumulation of secretions in the intertriginous spaces leads to maceration and necrotic decomposition on the surface, with the formation of malodorous material.
4. Malignant degeneration of condylomata acuminata is extremely rare (giant condylomata Buschke-Löwenstein).

Therapy

1. Podophyllin (25%) in alcoholic solution is helpful. The affected areas of the skin are dabbed with this solution 1 to 2 times per week. The healthy skin is covered with zinc paste to avoid irritation. After 30 minutes (vulva) or 4 to 6 hours (penis) a sitzbath is taken. Not more than 1 to 2 ml of this solution per day should be used to avoid podophyllin toxicity.
2. Large clusters of warts can be removed by electrocautery if podophyllin alone is insufficient.
3. The sexual partner should always be examined and treated if necessary to avoid ping pong infection.

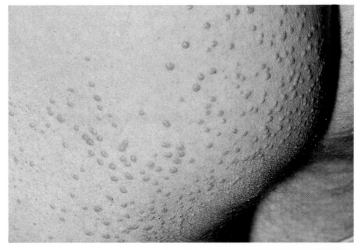

Figure 397. Eruptive xanthomas. Rapidly developing, yellowish to reddish lenticular tumors in the gluteal region.

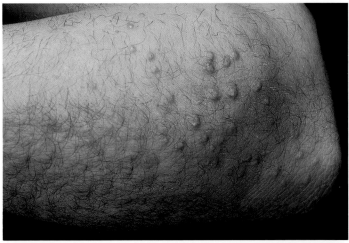

Figure 398. Eruptive xanthomas near the elbow.

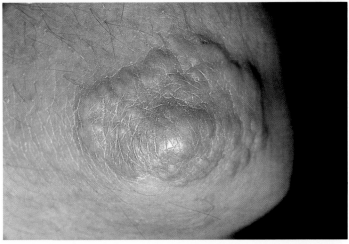

Figure 399. Tuberous xanthoma. Platelike tumor composed of yellowish nodules at the elbow.

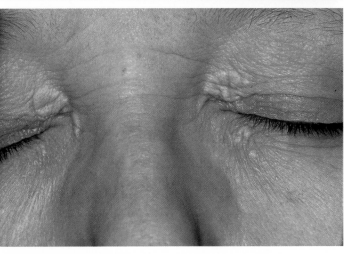

Figure 400. Xanthelasma palpebrarum. Slightly raised yellow-brown tumors at the medial corner of the eye.

Xanthoma, Xanthelasma

Eruptive Xanthomas

This is a genetically fixed, familial disturbance of fat metabolism (hyperlipidemia type I and IV and occasionally type V) that causes a dissemination of fat-storing tumors. The serum triglycerides are always increased. Lipid electrophoresis is necessary for exact classification.

Clinical Appearance

1. Pinhead to pea-sized yellow or pink nodules with a distinctly reddened basis are disseminated in large numbers. Nodules over the buttocks or the elbows occasionally coalesce.
2. Buttocks, chest, abdomen, back, arms, and face are mainly involved, rarely the oral mucosa (type I).
3. Frequent associated symptoms are hepatosplenomegaly and lipemia retinalis (type I) or obesity, diabetes mellitus, atherosclerosis, recurrent pancreatitis, and lipemia retinalis (type IV).

Therapy

Dietary measures are usually sufficient. Alcohol should be avoided; physical activity and weight reduction should be encouraged. Drug therapy is usually not necessary.

Tuberous Xanthomas

They are rare and belong to hyperlipidemia type II and occasionally types III and IV. They are often associated with hypercholesterinemia.

Clinical Appearance

1. Firm yellow or orange-red nodules with a diameter of 0.5 to 2.5 cm, and occasionally more, are characteristic. These nodules are often surrounded by a red halo. They do not cause any discomfort.
2. Knees and elbows are mainly affected; tumors may also be found on buttocks, heels, and palms.
3. Associated symptoms are xanthelasma palpebrarum and xanthomas of the tendons and fasciae. The cardiovascular system is frequently affected with myocardial infarction, intermittent claudication, arterial occlusive disease, cerebral hemorrhages, and so on. Involvement of the liver can lead to biliary cirrhosis. The gallbladder often contains cholesterin stones. Arcus cornealis ("arcus senilis") is sometimes a diagnostic sign of hypercholesterinemia.

Therapy

A low calorie, low cholesterol diet is helpful. Lipid-lowering medications such as Atromid-S are not always effective. Larger xanthomas may require surgical removal.

Xanthelasma Palpebrarum

Clinical Appearance

1. These frequent, easily recognizable changes in older people consist of soft, occasionally velvet-like, yellow nodules or plaques on the eyelids. They usually occur bilaterally and in symmetric fashion.
2. Xanthelasma is often found on the upper lid and in the inner canthus. They are also seen on the lower lid and, in extreme cases, involve the entire upper and lower lids.
3. In rare cases, a simultaneous hyperlipidemia exists with tuberous or eruptive xanthomas.

Therapy

Treatment is indicated only for cosmetic reasons. Excision under local anesthesia is the treatment of choice, but relapses occur frequently.

Part IV

Malignant Tumors and Potentially Malignant Tumors

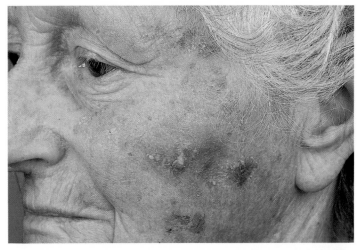

Figure 401. Actinic (solar) keratoses. Multiple, slightly raised hyperkeratotic, partly crust-covered areas in the face.

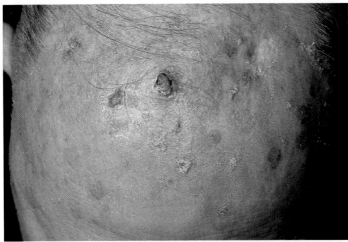

Figure 402. Actinic (solar) keratoses. Telangiectatic areas on the scalp with superimposed hyperkeratosis of varying degrees.

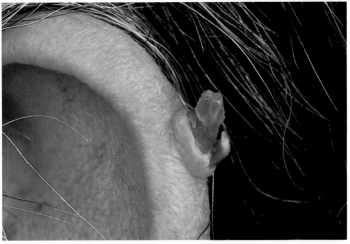

Figure 403. Cornu cutaneum on a keratoacanthoma. Cutaneous horn on a dish-shaped tumor of the auricular rim.

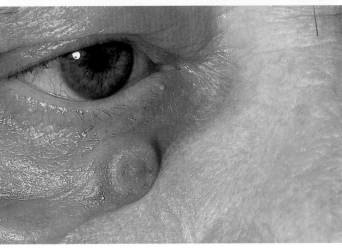

Figure 404. Keratoacanthoma. Round tumor with central pitting that is filled with a cornified cone.

Actinic Keratoses, Keratoacanthoma

Actinic Keratoses

Actinic or solar keratoses develop as a consequence of prolonged exposure to ultraviolet rays. They develop especially in older people and in people with open air occupations, such as farmers and seamen. Increasing exposure to UV light from changing recreational activities will gradually cause the incidence of these skin changes to increase, even in persons who are not exposed to sunlight through their occupations. Actinic keratoses must be taken seriously because they may represent a potential precursor stage to squamous cell carcinoma. This makes actinic keratoses more than just a cosmetic problem. Carcinomatous degeneration, however, does not occur very often and develops only after prolonged existence of the actinic keratosis.

Clinical Appearance

1. Initially, actinic keratoses are erythematous lesions of up to 1 cm in size. Their surface is covered with a crust of scales, which gives it a slightly rough consistency.
2. Some of these changes show increased pigmentation in some segments.
3. Occasionally the lesions are covered with thick keratinic layers with the appearance of a cutaneous horn (cornu cutaneum).
4. Increased infiltration of the base and beginning ulceration are an indication for diagnostic biopsy to rule out carcinomatous degeneration.

Therapy

1. In early cases, application of a fatty ointment (R.31a, b) and a sunscreen (see later) is sufficient.
2. Topical corticosteroids, sometimes in combination with urea or salicylic acid (R.37b, c), temporarily suppress the inflammatory reaction.
3. For topical treatment of advanced lesions, the cytostatic drug 5-fluorouracil is applied to the involved areas twice daily for 2 to 6 weeks until an erosive reaction occurs. (It should not be applied to the eyes, the nasolabial fold, or the oral region.) The surrounding healthy skin must be covered with a zinc paste.
4. The patient must be followed regularly until the lesions are healed.
5. All lesions suspected of malignancy must be biopsied; for smaller lesions an excisional biopsy is indicated.
6. Existing actinic damage of the skin cannot be reversed. The skin must be protected against light to avoid additional damage from UV exposure (hats with broad rim, sunscreen ointment with a high protective factor [R.43], no excessive exposure to sunlight).

Keratoacanthoma

Keratoacanthoma, a so-called pseudocarcinoma, occurs frequently and must be mentioned here. It is a solitary tumor that occurs in sun-exposed areas, especially in fair-skinned individuals. The tumor develops without pre-existing changes within a few weeks and disappears spontaneously after several months over a period of a few weeks or months. It usually leaves a shallow scar.

Clinical Appearance

A firm, skin-colored to red nodule of up to 2 cm in size with a horn-filled central crater that gradually increases is typical.

Therapy

The tumor is difficult to distinguish from a squamous cell carcinoma and should be excised for histologic examination.

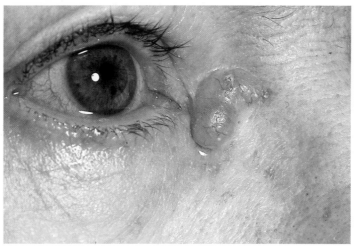

Figure 405. Basal cell epithelioma. Glassy-appearing tumor with superimposed enlarged blood vessels.

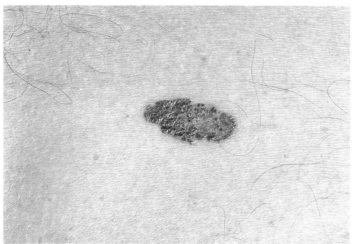

Figure 406. Pigmented basal cell epithelioma. Slightly raised tumor with marginal nodular seam and marked melanin pigmentation.

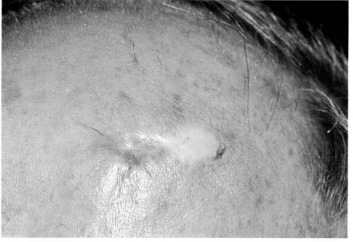

Figure 407. Morphealike basal cell epithelioma. White indurated region adjacent to an atrophic retracted area, similar to scar formation.

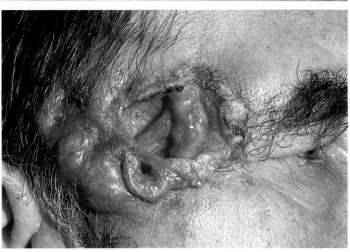

Figure 408. Basal cell epithelioma of the type ulcus terebrans. Extensive tumor in the temple area with destructive growth and deep ulcer formation.

Basal Cell Epithelioma (BCE)

A basal cell epithelioma seldom metastasizes but must be taken seriously because of its aggressive growth, with destruction of skin, cartilage, and bone. The fact that more than 80 per cent of all basal cell epitheliomas develop in the face plus their frequent occurrence in fair-skinned individuals in sunny areas (Australia, southern states of the United States) point to sunlight as an important factor. In addition, genetic factors and exposure to carcinogens, such as arsenic, may play a role. In more than 40 per cent of all patients, additional basal cell epitheliomas develop later.

Clinical Appearance

Five different types of basal cell epitheliomas can be distinguished on the basis of their different morphology.

1. *Nodular basal cell epithelioma*

   This is a skin-colored or somewhat lighter, transparent, soft nodule with overlying small telangiectasias. It grows slowly and may develop into a rodent ulcer after a growth period of up to several years.

2. *Rodent ulcer*

   With further growth, the blood supply to the central parts of the tumor becomes inadequate and central ulceration develops, with crust formation and occasional bleeding or weeping. The marginal nodules continue to grow and appear like a string of pearls. The overlying telangiectasias are typical for basal cell epithelioma.

3. *Ulcus terebrans*

   Development of most ulcerated basal cell epitheliomas remains restricted to the skin, but ulcus terebrans shows a very aggressive growth that can lead to significant destruction, especially in the face. The tumor can grow into the orbit and cause loss of eyesight. Life-threatening complications can occur when the skull is invaded (meningitis or massive hemorrhage caused by erosion of blood vessels).

4. *Pigmented basal cell epithelioma*

   This tumor has the same biologic behavior as other basal cell epitheliomas but in addition shows significant melanin pigmentation that occasionally can make it difficult to distinguish this tumor from malignant melanoma. It can be differentiated by its nodular margin, which is typical for basal cell epithelioma.

5. *Morphealike BCE*

   This tumor develops mainly in the face. Clinically, it has the appearance of a circumscribed, flat, occasionally slightly depressed lesion—like a scar. On close examination, it can be recognized as a basal cell epithelioma by the telangiectasias present in the tumor. These basal cell epitheliomas can be mistaken for scars for many years and sometimes grow to significant size; they can be difficult to manage.

Therapy

1. Operation. The extent of the operation depends on the size of the tumor. Procedures range from simple excisional biopsy to extensive excision with subsequent plastic surgery to cover the defect. The tissue surrounding the excised tumor must be examined histologically to confirm complete excision of the tumor. Basal cell epitheliomas, even small ones, must be excised well into normal tissue, with a "security distance" of at least 0.3 to 0.5 cm. Operative treatment has the advantage that complete removal of the tumor can be confirmed postoperatively by histologic examination. Operative procedures that result in complete tissue destruction, such as electrocurettage, are not recommended for treatment of basal cell epitheliomas.

2. Radiation therapy. In the hands of an experienced radiotherapist, the results with this treatment are as good as those obtained with operative procedures. The diagnosis must be confirmed by biopsy before treatment is started. Today, radiotherapy is recommended for elderly patients (more than 70 years) with extensive tumors who present an increased operative risk. Ten to twenty radiation treatments are required; they are followed by an inflammatory reaction for several weeks. The cosmetic result is initially good but may deteriorate later. This treatment carries the risk of a roentgen carcinoma 10 to 20 years later.

3. The patients must be seen annually for follow-up examinations of the involved areas, especially those exposed to light.

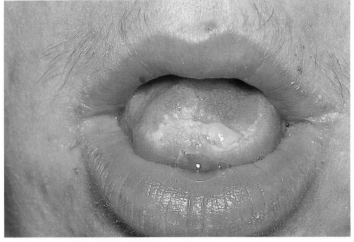

Figure 409. Leukoplakia. White hyperkeratosis of the tongue with poorly defined borders.

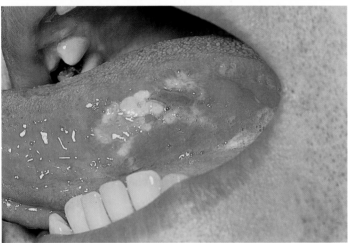

Figure 410. Leukoplakia-like Bowen's disease on the rim of the tongue. Partly erosive and partly leukoplakia-like tumor with irregular margins.

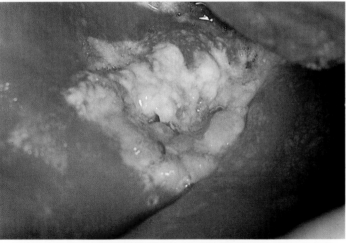

Figure 411. Leukoplakia carcinoma on the buccal mucosa. Diffuse leukoplakia with indistinct margins. A markedly hyperkeratotic infiltrating carcinoma is visible in the center of the lesion.

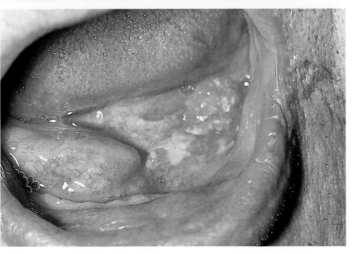

Figure 412. Leukoplakia-like Bowen's disease of the floor of the mouth. Diffuse, partly erosive, partly leukoplakia-like tumor with indistinct margins.

Leukoplakia

Leukoplakia is a plaquelike lesion occurring on the red of the lips or the oral or genital mucosa. Most of these are benign and do not require tumor-specific treatment. About 10 per cent of leukoplakias must be regarded as potentially precancerous lesions; a carcinoma in situ is hidden in approximately 3 per cent. Occasionally, one may find widespread carcinomatous changes in a leukoplakia (leukoplakia-carcinoma). In some cases of mucosal carcinoma, leukoplakia may be present on the surface from the beginning or develop there later, for instance in Bowen's disease. Leukoplakia develops frequently from mechanical irritation (defective teeth, poorly fitting dentures), from chemical irritation (smoking), or in hereditary or acquired diseases, such as virus papilloma, mucosal lichen planus (see p. 87), white sponge nevus, and dyskeratosis congenita. Consultation with an experienced stomatologist may be indicated.

Clinical Appearance

1. A sharply delineated, occasionally raised, white patch or indurated white plaque is characteristic, occasionally with erosions and a knobby or verrucous surface.
2. It is often located in the corner of the mouth, but the entire oral mucosa can be involved.
3. Irregular, spotty leukoplakia lesions on an erythematous base or lesions with erosions, ulcerations, and irregular, exophytic growth are always suspicious for carcinomatous changes.

Therapy

1. Treatment is unnecessary, if the cause of the mucosal irritation is known and can be avoided. In these cases, the leukoplakia usually disappears with time after the irritation has been removed. Smoking should be stopped and dentures repaired. The patient must be seen for followup examination at regular intervals until the lesion is healed.
2. Local application of Vitamin A solution can occasionally effect healing.
3. Long-term treatment of pre-invasive leukoplakia with Etretinate (R.59) has now been proved as effective.
4. In cases without recognizable cause or leukoplakias that do not heal within 4 to 6 weeks with the previous measures or those in which carcinoma is suspected, the entire lesion should be excised as soon as possible. Lesions too large for total excision can be treated with excision of the suspicious area. If histologic examination reveals malignant degeneration, the tumor should be treated with more radical procedures such as wide excision, neck dissection, or radiation therapy.

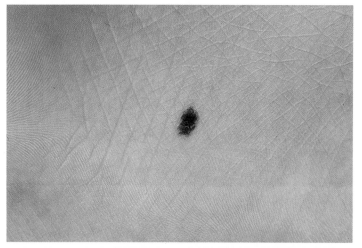

Figure 413. Nevus-cell nevus. Signs of proliferation with dysplasia clinically recognizable by its ragged, partly indistinct margin.

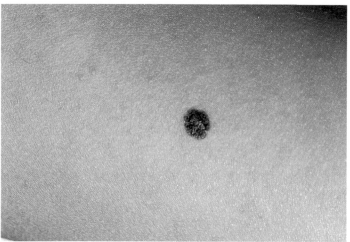

Figure 414. Nevus-cell nevus. Polycyclic margins and black-brown pigmentation as a sign of increased proliferation.

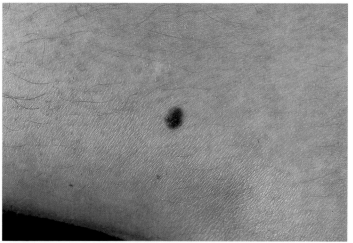

Figure 415. Superficial spreading melanoma. These early cases are often difficult to distinguish from a nevus-cell nevus by appearance alone.

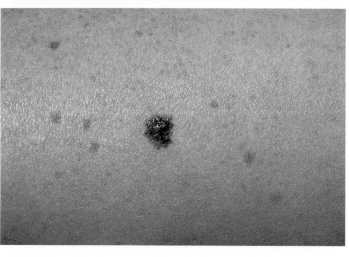

Figure 416. Early superficial spreading melanoma. Polycyclic margins, heterogenous pigmentation, slightly raised in the darker parts.

Malignant Melanoma

The incidence of this extremely malignant tumor has increased three- to fourfold in the last 20 years. In some patients, especially those with fair skin, excessive exposure to sunlight may be a factor. Patients with previous primary melanoma in the history and those who have family members with malignant melanoma are especially prone to develop malignant melanoma.

It is extremely important to recognize the tumor as early as possible; the patient's chance of survival is much better with early treatment. The prognosis depends on the size of the tumor and its depth. The attending physician must be familiar with the early signs of malignant degeneration and should refer the patient immediately for competent evaluation and treatment.

Premalignant Changes and Early Types of Malignancy

In the early stage, as long as the tumor is only a few millimeters in size, it can be very difficult to differentiate a melanoma from a nevus-cell nevus, especially from a "dysplastic nevus-cell nevus." These are regarded as potential precursors of malignant melanoma. They show marked pigmentation and have ragged edges. Histologic examination reveals cell dysplasia of varying degrees. More than 80 per cent of malignant melanomas occur on apparently normal skin. A few develop in benign nevus-cell nevi but they are exceptions.

Small pigmented tumors must be regarded as suspicious when the following criteria are present:

1. Rapid growth over a period of a few weeks or months
2. Changes in pigmentation; especially darker discoloration; central hypo- or hyperpigmentation; grey, blue, or red discoloration within the tumor
3. Inflammatory red margin
4. Ragged borders

Other very suspicious signs in small and especially in larger tumors are

5. weeping, crust formation
6. bleeding, spontaneously or with minimal trauma
7. itching.

All these symptoms are only suspicious signs and can also occur in traumatized or "active" nevus-cell nevi. One-time or repeated trauma to a nevus-cell nevus does not induce development of a malignant melanoma. Injury to a malignant melanoma, however, could cause it to metastasize. Lymphogenic cutaneous satellite tumors in the vicinity of the lesion are not just a suspicious sign but confirm the presence of a malignant melanoma.

The differential diagnosis, early forms included, should consider pigmented nevus and many other skin tumors such as angiokeratoma, pigmented basal cell epithelioma, seborrheic keratosis, pyogenic granuloma, and so on. Consultation with an experienced dermatologist/oncologist may be indicated. Melanosis circumscripta praeblastomatosa (lentigo maligna) is another of the early malignant types of melanoma (see p. 217). Treatment in the "freckle" stage usually results in a cure rate of 100 per cent.

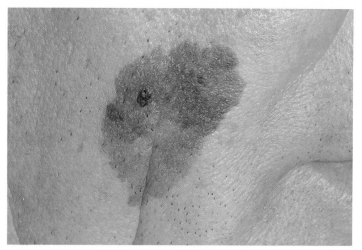

Figure 417. Lentigo maligna (melanosis circumscripta praeblastomatosa Dubreuilh). Well-defined, heterochromic pigmentation of the skin with notched borders.

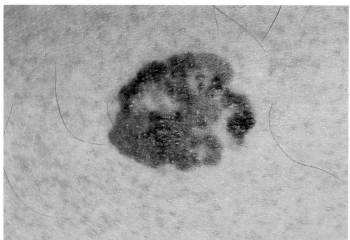

Figure 418. Superficial spreading melanoma. Slightly raised tumor with notched borders and mainly dark brown pigmented nodules as well as depigmented areas of regression.

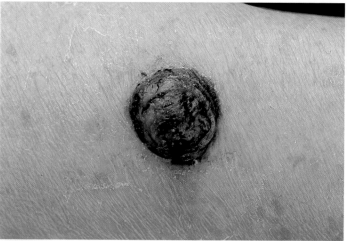

Figure 419. Nodular melanoma. Round, nodular, sharply delineated black tumor with easily traumatized surface.

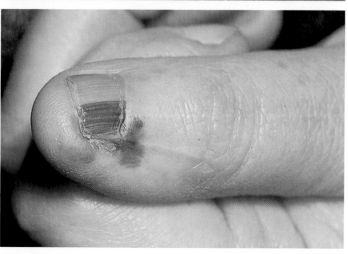

Figure 420. Acral lentiginous melanoma. Horizontal, not yet nodular growth phase. Irregular pigmentation adjacent to the nail, partly extending into the nail plate.

Clinical Types of Melanoma

Clinical Appearance

Four different types of malignant melanoma can be distinguished:

Superficial Spreading Melanoma (SSM) (approximately 70 per cent of all melanomas)
Initially the tumor presents itself in its superficial form for several months up to a few years and grows at a moderate speed. It is a flat tumor with a notched border and usually consists of many small nodules. .Individual central or marginal areas show signs of regression and are skin colored or have a reddish or bluish (from deep-seated pigment remnants) color. Later, nodular or erosive changes occur in parts of the tumor, indicating a poorer prognosis (greater maximal thickness of the tumor). Superficial spreading melanomas are found mainly on trunk and extremities.

Nodular Melanoma (NM) (16 per cent of all melanomas)
This is a dark brown to black pigmented tumor that grows vertically and horizontally in a nodular fashion. Mild trauma causes bleeding or weeping. The tumor metastasizes rapidly and has a poor prognosis. Amelanotic tumors are sometimes observed. Nodular melanomas occur mainly on the trunk and the extremities.

Lentigo Maligna Melanoma (LMM) (Melanoma on melanosis circumscripta praeblastomatosa) (5 per cent of all melanomas)
This tumor occurs almost exclusively in the face, usually in older people and on skin injured by excessive exposure to light. It is a sharply or poorly demarcated, homogenous tumor with varying degrees of light to dark brown discoloration. The lesion is level with the surrounding skin (melanosis circumscripta praeblastomatosa). After 5 to 15 years, a tumorous nodule develops on this lesion that may show zones of regression like those seen in superficial spreading melanomas. Then, the prognosis is poor.

Acral-Lentiginous Melanoma (ALM) (5 to 10 per cent of all melanomas)
This also is a tumor that grows horizontally for some time and presents itself as an enlarging patch. The typical location of this tumor is on the hands and feet, occasionally subungual or in the skin surrounding the nails.

Unclassifiable Melanomas (UCM)
Approximately 3 to 4 per cent of all melanomas do not fall into these categories.
Local metastases into the surrounding skin and the regional lymph nodes as well as distant metastases characterize the later stages.

Therapy

Each tumor suspicious for melanoma should be evaluated by a dermatologist experienced in oncology before treatment is started because many other skin tumors must be considered in the differential diagnosis. Incisional or punch biopsies should be avoided if at all possible.

Subsequent therapy should be performed in a department of dermatology with the necessary expertise in the treatment of these tumors. The primary tumor, provided no metastases are present, should be excised well into healthy tissue.

Surgery is the treatment of choice; all operable tumors should be excised. Mutilating surgery in advanced melanoma cannot be recommended. Chemotherapy (DTIC) is used to treat melanomas of clinical stage III (distant metastases). In general, this is not very effective but can occasionally show surprising results in individual patients. Up-to-date results of immunologic therapy have been disappointing. Follow-up examinations at 3- to 6-month intervals are necessary after treatment is completed.

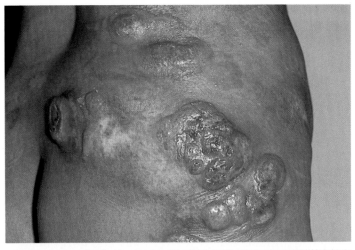

Figure 421. Cutaneous T-cell lymphoma, mycosis fungoides, and multiple, ulcerating tumors.

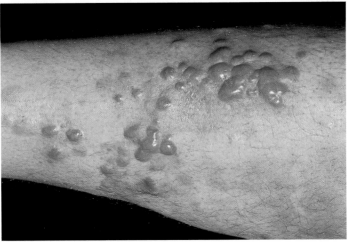

Figure 422. Cutaneous B-cell lymphoma. Rapidly developing, firm, partly glassy-appearing small tumors, lower leg.

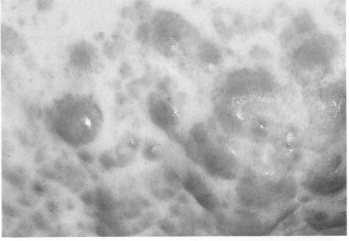

Figure 423. Malignant lymphoma (immunocytoma) of the skin. Densely arranged tumors in various stages of development.

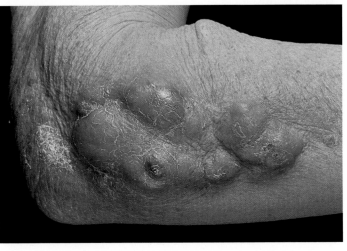

Figure 424. Centroblastic malignant lymphoma of the skin. Nodular, firm aggregate of tumors.

Mycosis Fungoides and Other Malignant Lymphomas

The term "malignant lymphomas" includes many diseases characterized by malignant proliferation of lymphocytes. A thorough knowledge of the early symptoms is important for the practicing physician. The first signs of the disease can be skin tumors and generalized symptoms such as fatigue, malaise, and increasing weight loss, which may lead to cachexia, as well as symptoms caused by the space-occupying growth of intestinal malignant lymphomas in lymph nodes, spleen, or bone marrow. The lymph nodes can be enlarged and palpable, as in chronic lymphatic leukemia. Depending on the degree of malignancy, the disease can last for months or years. Early diagnosis and treatment can often produce long-term remissions or even cures.

Malignant lymphoma can affect the skin as a primary or secondary (metastatic) tumor. With primary skin involvement, the disease can often be limited to the skin for years, especially with mycosis fungoides, less often with other malignant lymphomas.

Pseudolymphomas are lymphocytic inflammatory reactions due to a number of different causes (Borrelia infections, analgesics) that can resemble malignant lymphomas clinically and histologically. They disappear completely after some time (for instance lymphocytoma, see p. 55).

Clinical Appearance

Mycosis Fungoides

The precursor stage consists of uncharacteristic itching and eczematous, widespread plaques and may last for several years. It is followed by tumorous infiltrates and nodules in the skin. The disease may last for 5 to 10 years or even longer. Mycosis fungoides is regarded as malignant lymphoma of low malignancy.

Other Malignant Lymphomas

Individual or multiple red to brown-red or blue-red, often ulcerating, nodules or nodular infiltrates are typical skin lesions. The tumors can remain restricted to the skin for some time before internal organs become involved. Frequently, only one or a few nodules are present and can regress with treatment. After a remission of weeks, months, or even years, the tumors usually recur. Among these solitary or multiple malignant lymphomas, one distinguishes lymphomas of high and low grade malignancy. In rare cases, malignant lymphoma manifests itself as disseminated multiple small tumors involving the entire skin. In these patients, the disease runs a rapid course with a fatal outcome within a few months (malignant lymphoma of high malignancy).

Therapy

Lasting cures are rare in patients with malignant lymphoma and skin manifestations, but long-lasting remissions can occasionally be achieved with appropriate therapeutic measures. An exact classification according to histologic and immunocytologic criteria should be attempted before treatment is started.

1. Malignant lymphomas of the skin are sensitive to radiation, especially low voltage therapy and fast electrons.
2. PUVA therapy can also produce long-lasting remission of mycosis fungoides.
3. Treatment with cytostatic drugs and corticosteroids can lead to partial and complete remission and is used in different combinations and in cyclic fashion depending on the degree of malignancy and the clinical stage of the disease. This treatment should be performed by a dermatologist or a hematologist with experience in oncologic therapy.

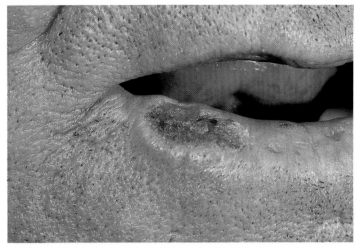

Figure 425. Squamous cell carcinoma of the lower lip. Centrally ulcerated tumor with a firm, raised margin.

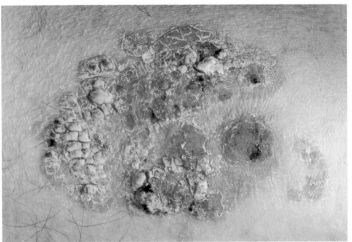

Figure 426. Bowen's disease. Flat, partly hyperkeratotic, partly erosive tumor, resembling psoriasis. The tumor developed over a period of several years.

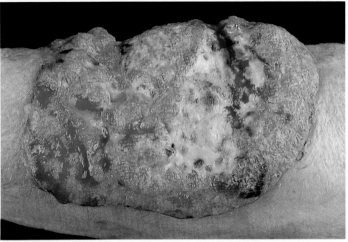

Figure 427. Squamous cell carcinoma of the forearm. Exophytic tumor with necrotic surface.

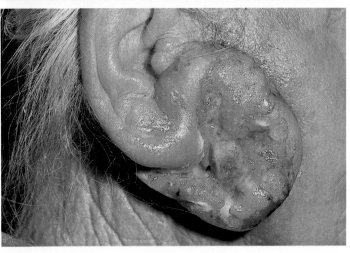

Figure 428. Squamous cell carcinoma of the ear. Ulcerating tumor, infiltrating the auricle.

Squamous Cell Carcinoma

This tumor usually occurs on skin damaged by chronic exposure to ionizing radiation (sunlight, x-rays) or carcinogens (tar, arsenic). It rarely develops on the basis of chronic inflammation (lupus vulgaris, chronic leg ulcer) or on contracted scars. The latent period after exposure to the causative agent can be several decades for arsenic or x-rays. With prompt treatment, squamous cell carcinomas can often be cured. The cure rate for small squamous cell carcinomas (up to 3 cm) is more than 90 per cent. Squamous cell carcinoma originating from precancerous lesions such as actinic keratoses grows very slowly and therefore is often neglected for quite some time. Metastases are seen especially in neglected cases or in carcinomas of lips, vulva, anus, or penis and in carcinomas of the oral cavity. Squamous cell carcinomas developing on skin damaged by light exposure have a relatively good prognosis. One must keep in mind, however, that these patients can later develop other carcinomas on their damaged skin.

Clinical Appearances

1. Initial changes appear as chronic eczema-like lesions with discrete, slowly increasing keratinization.
2. With endophytic growth, an ulcer develops with a firm wall and papillomatous changes in the ulcer, whereas a more exophytic growth will lead to a raised papillary-verrucous tumor with a thick horny surface, occasionally with the appearance of a cutaneous horn. Long-standing squamous cell carcinomas occasionally have a friable, weeping, or bleeding surface.
3. Necrotic changes in the tumor and bacterial infection can produce malodorous crusts.
4. Palpable, firm swelling of the regional lymph nodes is an indication that the tumor has metastasized.

Therapy

1. The treatment of choice at this time is operative removal of the tumor and histologic examination to confirm complete removal of the pathologic tissue. Extensive tumors may require biopsy to determine the stage of the tumor, the degree of cell differentiation, and how radical the operative procedure must be. Radical operative procedures with removal of the regional lymph nodes may be indicated for tumors with poor prognosis due to location.
2. Patients who are high operative or anesthesia risks may be better treated with radiation therapy (x-rays, fast electrons, or gamma rays).
3. Cytostatic drugs, especially bleomycin, are used to reduce the size of the tumor preoperatively (ENT tumors) and when metastases are present.
4. Occasionally, one finds inoperable, widespread squamous cell carcinomas, especially in old patients. These tumors can only be treated with palliative measures (pain control, palliative radiation).
5. Regular tumor follow-up is necessary for early detection of recurrences, metastases, or newly formed tumors.

Part V

Selected Commercial Preparations and Prescriptions with Practical Guidelines for Treatment

General Principles

This chapter describes a selection of topical and systemic medications we have found useful for treatment of the skin diseases covered in this book. For reasons of clarity, only a few representative preparations are discussed for each group. Similar specialities can be used in a similar manner. Many skin diseases can be treated either with local or with systemic medications. Topical treatment, however, is preferable in most cases, because the lesions are reached more effectively by the active medication and the systemic effects on the body are less pronounced than they would be with internal therapy.

More than 1000 special preparations are available for topical treatment alone. The total number of systemic and topical medications for treatment of skin diseases is so great that a certain selection must be made to allow the practicing physician to be familiar with the indications, limitations, and side effects of the drugs of choice.

Compounding of medications is used very rarely today in most fields of medicine with the exception of dermatology. The practice has become discredited by the questionable use of outmoded, ineffective, and harmful drugs. This is regrettable, because some formulations are quite useful in practice.

Topical preparations usually consist of bases that contain the active drugs, and occasionally additives. The following preparations are in use as bases or vehicles:

A. Moist dressings (see p. 227)
B. Partial and full baths (see p. 227)
C. Powders (see p. 228)
D. Solutions, tinctures (see p. 228)
E. Shake mixtures (see p. 229)
F. Gels (see p. 230)
G. Pastes (see p. 230)
H. Emulsions, creams, ointments (see p. 231)

Contrary to systemic therapy, where the vehicle is used only to enhance solubility or to act as a carrier substance (vehicle or base), it also has important pharmacologic effects when used for topical treatment. These effects can be on either a physical or a chemical basis. The therapeutic effect of powders and shake mixtures, for instance, depends almost exclusively on physical properties (they increase the effective surface, act as hygroscopic agents, reduce friction in moist body folds, and so on), but delivery of the active medication to the skin is poor.

On the other hand, pharmacologically active ingredients dissolve well in cream and ointment bases and in alcohol (tinctures) and are released at the site of application.

Today, rational treatment must include pharmacologic as well as economic considerations. The following points must be taken into account.

1. In addition to the effective drug, many commercial preparations contain other chemicals that are unnecessary. They may make the medication more expensive and can even cause undesired side effects (i.e., contact eczema). The physician must decide whether all the components of a particular preparation are necessary for the desired therapeutic effect. Medications with only one active drug are preferred, since treatment with combined preparations is less flexible.
2. For everyday practice, it is important to accurately inform the patient about the following: the areas of the skin to be treated, how often the topical therapy must be carried out, and how long treatment will be continued. Precise information regarding these points tends to improve the therapeutic result and to reduce the cost of treatment.
3. Another important point is to prescribe an appropriate amount of the effective drug. Small amounts are relatively more expensive than larger quantities. For a limited dermatosis (such as acute contact dermatitis), the prescription of a small tube can be quite economic. For chronic skin diseases, the prescribed amount should be sufficient to allow the patient to carry out adequate topical treatment until the next office visit.

The following are rough estimates of the amounts necessary to treat different areas of the skin. The amounts given are for ointments. For creams, the amounts have to be increased by 10 to 30 per cent. For a lotion, the amount should be doubled.

Table 1

Treated area	Amount for one treatment (gm)	Amount for 14 days, for application twice daily (gm)
Hands, face	2	50
Anogenital area	2	50
One arm, chest, or back	3	80
One leg	4	120
Entire body	25–40	approximately 1000

4. A thin application of a cream or an ointment is usually sufficient. Application of a thick layer does not increase the effectiveness of the active ingredient because its resorption is not dependent on the thickness of the applied layer. By "treating" the clothing it only increases the amount of medication used. It is possible, however, to force penetration of drug remnants that have remained on the surface by saturating the skin with fat. This can be done by applying an ointment containing the effective drug in the morning and an ointment without the effective drug in the evening.

5. With expensive corticosteroid preparations, a so-called interval therapy can be used. This alternates periods of therapy with drug-containing preparations with periods of therapy with drug-free preparations in intervals of 2 to 3 days. With this program, the effect can be even better, because cortisone tachyphylaxis can be avoided. Treatment is more cost effective and cortisone side effects occur less frequently.

6. Compounding medications can also be less expensive. Mixing standard (U.S.P.) bases with commercial preparations is not recommended, however. Commercial preparations are often complicated emulsions that can become unstable when mixed, and they usually become more expensive when processed further in a pharmacy. On the other hand, prescriptions with U.S.P. bases and active medications have the advantage that they are free of preservatives. It is preferable for the primary care physician to limit the use of these prescriptions to a few preparations until she or he is thoroughly familiar with them.

Medications and Measures for External Treatment

A. Wet Dressings

They are anti-inflammatory, cooling, and desiccating and are helpful for weeping, erosive, or ulcerative lesions. They can be used to debride wounds by cleansing the skin of crusts and exudates and by helping to maintain drainage of affected sites.

Application: Use several layers of moist gauze or pieces of linen (wick effect), renew every 20 minutes. (Caution: Prolonged use can lead to maceration.)

R.1. Bland, anti-inflammatory:
Tap water
Physiologic saline solution
The addition of alcohol (isopropyl, 1:5 to 1:10) produces increased cooling, drying, and degreasing.
Aluminum subacetate solution (Burow's solution) 1:20 to 1:40 is astringent and may be used on oozing or vesicular sites.

R.2. Antibacterial:
Silver nitrate (0.1–0.5%), $KMnO_4$ (1:1000 to 1:10,000)

B. Partial Baths (Hand Bath, Footbath, Sitzbath) and Full Baths

They are anti-inflammatory and drying.

R.3. Bland, soothing:
Add colloidal substances such as Linit or corn starch. Add a handful of the substance to the running bath water. (Prepared colloid bath products such as Aveeno or Oilated Aveeno are available.)

R.4. Disinfectant:
Add $KMnO_4$ until the bath water is a pale purple. (1:25,000)

R.5. Degreasing:
Acetone 1:20 or alcohol 1:10 is helpful for localized areas; Sebanil, Ionax skin cleanser.

R.6. Antiscaling:
Soft soap

R.7. Bath oils:
Alpha Keri
Domol
Lubath
Surfol

R.8. Toughening the skin:
Salicylic acid (1–2%) is a keratoplastic agent that tends to increase the thickness of the horny layer. In Europe, a tannic acid solution (oak bark extract) would be used. Tannic acid solution may be made by infusing four tea bags in a quart of water.

R.9. Antipruritic, anti-inflammatory:
Tar preparations such as Balnetar (2.5%), Polytar (25%), Zetar emulsion (30%).

R.10. Shampoos:
    a. Antiseborrheic: Ionil T, Sebutone, T/Gel, Vanseb T
    b. Antiseborrheic-antimicrobial: Zincon, DHS—Zinc, Danex

C. Powders

Powders have a drying effect and decrease friction. This makes them very useful to keep skinfolds such as the groin, axillae, and the submammary area dry. Active medications are released from powders to a lesser degree than from other vehicles.

R.11. Nonmedicated (or inert):
    Talc
    Cornstarch
    Zinc oxide or stearate

R.12. Anti-infectious:
    Polymyxin powder
    Hexachlorophene powder
    Bacitracin powder

R.13. Antimycotics:
    Micatin: Miconazole powder
    Tinactin: Tolnaftate powder (effective against dermatophytes only)
    Mycostatin: Nystatin powder (effective against yeasts only)
    Desenex: Undecylenic acid powder

D. Solutions, Tinctures

Mixtures of pharmacologic agents with water (solutions) or alcohol (tinctures) or alcohol in conjunction with polyethylene glycol have a desiccating and defatting effect. After evaporation of the solvent, the effective substance remains on the skin. These are very useful for the hairy parts of the head, the interdigital areas of the foot, and the intertriginous areas.

R.14. Antimycotic, antibacterial:
    a. Dyes
       • Castellani's paint (Carbol-fuchsin solution)
       • Gentian violet (0.1–0.5%) (Caution: Danger of necrosis when applied in
         intertriginous areas in concentrations higher than 0.5%.)
    b. Tolnaftate: Tinactin solution (effective against dermatophytes only)
    c. Clotrimazole U.S.P.: Lotrimin solution; Mycelex solution
       Miconazole: Micatin solution
       Haloprogin: Halotex solution

R.15. Antiviral:
    Idoxuridine (IDUR): Stoxil (not available in U.S.)
    Trifluridine: Viroptic ophthalmic solution.

R.16. Anti-inflammatory, anti-infectious (tar-containing preparations):

    a. Crude coal tar solution (liquor carbonis detergens, LCD), 2–5%

    b. Arning's tincture

        Rx: Anthrarobin   1.0

            Tumenol   4.0

            Tinct. Benzoes   10.0

            Aether. sulf. ad 30.0

R.17. Disinfectant:

Mercurochrome solution (Caution: Rare allergy to mercury.)

    Advantage: Burning after application is minimal.

Thimerosal (merthiolate) (Caution: Allergy to mercury possible.)

Betadine solution (povidone-iodine)

Iodine 2% and sodium iodine 2.4% (solution, tincture) (Caution: Allergy to iodine possible.)

R.18. Scalp tinctures (anti-inflammatory, contain corticosteroids):

Benecort topical solution (1%–2½% hydrocortisone)

Synalar solution (0.01% fluocinolone acetonide)

Lidex solution (0.5% fluocinonide)

R.19. Antihidrotic:

    a. Rx: Aluminum chloride 20.0–30.0

            Aqua dest. ad 100.0

            Apply in the evening, leave for 15 minutes, then rinse off.

    b. Drysol (20% aluminum chloride solution)

        Use: Apply overnight 2 times and then once or twice weekly.

E. Shake Mixtures

Combination of solid and liquid materials—"liquid powder." Effect similar to that of powders: anti-inflammatory, desiccating, cooling, better adherence, especially to large areas. Shake mixtures contain much water but little or no oil, not suitable for dry skin. As in powders, the effect is mainly through physical properties. There is little or no release of active medications.

R.20. Inert:

    a. Drying

        Nonalcoholic white shake lotion:

        Rx: zinc oxide   20 gm

            talcum   20 gm

            glycerin   30 gm

            distilled water qs ad 100 ml

    b. Strong drying effect

        Alcoholic white shake lotion:

        Rx: zinc oxide   15 gm

            talcum   15 gm

            glycerin   10 gm

            95% alcohol   30 ml

            distilled water qs ad 100 ml

    c. Commercial preparation with similar effect

        Calamine lotion (antipruritic)

R.21. Strong anti-inflammatory effect:
Triamcinolone (Volon A Shake mixture); not commercially available in the United States.

R.22. Antibacterial:
Rivanol (1%)-zinc shake mixture; not commercially available in the United States.

F. Gels

A base (usually propylene glycol) with high water content has a cooling and antipruritic effect. Alcoholic gels have a drying effect and may cause skin irritation, especially when the skin is dry.

R.23. Cooling, anesthetizing, antipruritic:
Topical gel (contains menthol, camphor, and benzyl alcohol)
Anbesol Gel (contains benzocaine, for use on or around the lips or in the mouth)

R.24. Acne medication:
Benzoyl peroxide has sebostatic, keratolytic, and antibacterial effects.
  (Caution: contact allergies and irritation are possible.)
  3–5% gel for the face; 10% for the trunk
Tretinoin (Vitamin A acid) has keratolytic and sebostatic effects.
  (Caution: Increased photosensitivity and skin irritation!)
  a. Benzoyl peroxide
    Desquam X
    Benzac W   } Aqueous gel base
    Panoxyl AQ
    Panoxyl: Alcohol gel base
    Benzac: Alcohol gel base   } More drying effect
    Persa-Gel: Acetone gel base
  b. Vitamin A
    Retin A gel 0.01% and 0.025%
Gels are used most frequently, but low fat emulsions are also useful for very sensitive skin (R.42).

R.25. Antimycotic:
Naftifin: Exoderil gel; not commercially available in the United States.
Bifonazol: Mycospor gel
Tolnaftate: Aftate gel (selectively against dermatophytes)

R.26. Antiparasitic:
Lindane and benzyl benzoate: Jacutin Gel

G. Pastes

These consist of powder components incorporated into an ointment. They are indicated for acute inflammatory dermatoses where desiccation and bland protective coating are desired. Pastes are not frequently used and there are few commercially made.

R.27. Bland coating:
Zinc oxide paste (USP) (Lassar's)
Rx: zinc oxide   25.0
     starch   25.0
     white petrolatum to make 100.0

R.28. Moderate coating effect:

Soft zinc paste

Rx:	zinc oxide	30.0
	olive oil	20.0
	lanolin to make 100.0	

R.29. Antimycotic:

Nystatin: Candio Hermal Paste   Effective against yeasts only.
                Multilind Paste   These preparations are
                Myco-Intradermi Paste   available in Europe.

R.30. Anti-inflammatory, antieczematous:

a. Tumenol-zinc paste:

Rx:	Tumenol-ammonium	5.0
	talc	25.0
	zinc oxide	25.0
	white petrolatum to make 100.0	

b. Coal tar distillate 5%: tarpaste

c. Locacorten vioform paste (combination of the antimicrobial dye vioform with a corticosteroid; available in Europe)

H. Emulsions: Lotions, Creams, Ointments

Lotions or creams are emulsions of the milk type (oil in water). Ointments are emulsions of either the butter type (water in oil) or completely water-free and occasionally even water-repellent bases (petrolatum, paraffin). A water-free but washable base, for instance, is polyethylene glycol ointment, a so-called lipogel. These bases are often used in commercial preparations because of their good release of active medications. Preparations with a higher fat content irritate the skin more, and the occlusive effect increases. Lotions and creams are unstable and usually contain a significant amount of additives (preservatives, emulsifiers, stabilizers) that can, in rare instances, cause reactions of intolerance.

On the other hand, patients usually find creams and lotions more pleasant than ointments. It must be kept in mind that with increasing water content, the quantity of topical medication necessary also increases (p. 226).

R.31. Preparations without active medications for interval therapy, for treatment of dry skin, and for skin protection:

a. Very strong lubricating effect
     White petrolatum, USP
     Mineral oil, liquid paraffin

b. Strong lubricating effect
     Hydrophilic petrolatum USP
     Eucerin
     Keri cream
     Nivea

c. Mild lubricating effect
     Hydrophilic ointment, USP
     Aquacare
     Lubriderm
     Purpose cream
     Moisturelle
     Cold cream USP (rose water ointment)

d. Cooling and mildly lubricating
     Sarna lotion
     Dermassage lotion

R.32. Antibacterial:

Antibiotics are used much too often for topical therapy. Topical antibiotics are indicated only in rare cases. Their use may lead to the development of resistance and contact sensitization.

The following discussion does not cover preparations containing antibiotics *that are indispensable* for systemic treatment (e.g., gentamicin) or related drugs that can produce cross-resistance or contact allergies (neomycin). The wide use of topical antibiotics in acne is not recommended.

Meclocycline: Meclan cream
Bacitracin: Bacitracin ointment
Chlortetracycline: Aureomycin ointment
Polymyxin B-Bacitracin: Polysporin ointment
Povidone-iodine: Betadine ointment
Clioquinol: Vioform cream, ointment; Torofor cream

R.33. Antimycotic:

a. Miconazole: Micatin,
   Monistat-Derm
   Econazole: Spectazole
   Haloprogin: Halotex
   Clotrimazole: Lotrimin,
   Mycelex

Broad-spectrum antimycotics effective against yeasts and dermatophytes

b. Tolnaftate: Tinactin cream (selectively against dermatophytes)
c. Nystatin: Mycostatin or Nilstat
   Effective against yeast only
d. Amphotericin B: Fungizone

R.34. Antiviral:

Acyclovir: Zovirax ointment

R.35. Antipsoriatic:

Preparations containing Dithranol (Cignolin, Anthralin)

Anthralin causes dermatitis of the nonaffected skin. Concentration of the active medication should be increased slowly until the optimal dose is reached. (Caution: Irritation with high concentration.) The ointment must not be applied to the face. Oxidation products of this substance can cause permanent discoloration of clothing.

Lasan Creams 0.1, 0.2, 0.4, 1%
Anthra-Derm ointment 0.1, 0.25, 0.5, 1%
Lasan unguent 0.4% anthralin
Drithocreme 0.1, 0.25, 0.5, 1%
Anthralin in a vanishing cream base
Formulations with Anthralin that are compounded should be dispensed in graded
   concentrations of 0.05 to 2%, preferably in white petrolatum with the addition
   of 2% salicylic acid (protects from oxidation).

R.36. Corticosteroids:

They are the most effective substances for topical anti-inflammatory therapy. To avoid undesirable cortisone side effects, it is better to use short-term or interval therapy with more potent cortisone preparations rather than continuous long-term therapy with less potent preparations (attenuation of the cortisone effect by tachyphylaxis). The dispensation of commercial preparations diluted with an indifferent base is especially inexpedient in this regard. Long-term (more than 6 weeks; depending on the potency) or excessive use of topical corticosteroids can cause undesirable side effects, such as epidermal and dermal atrophy, local hypertrichosis, development of telangiectasias, steroid rosacea of the face, enhancement of infections, and striae. All but the latter may be reversible. They occur specially with prolonged application of corticosteroid preparations to areas of thin skin (eyelids, face, genitals) or intertriginous areas such as the axillae, groin, and submammary region. Ocular hypertension may occur from application in or around the eyes.

Some of the cortisone applied to the skin is absorbed and can produce systemic cortisone effects, especially with application of potent corticosteroids over large areas of the body (more than 25 per cent of the body surface). Systemic side effects are more likely to occur in infants and children than in adults, and if used in areas of good absorption (intertriginous skin).

Penetration of the drug is enhanced by hydration of the skin and by application under occlusive plastic gloves, shower cap, household plastic wrap, and so on, fixed with tight-fitting clothing or tubegauze dressings. Occlusion promotes desirable as well as undesirable effects of cortisone.

The effect of corticosteroid preparations depends on the concentration as well as on the selected drug. For practical purposes, corticosteroids can be divided into weak, medium, and strong preparations. Weak preparations should be used for thin skin (face, infants) and in skin folds.

    a. Relatively weak cortisone preparations
        Hydrocortisone 1% cream and ointment
        Generic
        Hytone
        Nutracort (lotion and cream)
        Synacort cream
        Desonide 0.05%: Tridesilon cream

    b. Corticosteroid preparations of medium strength
        Triamcinolone 0.1% cream: Kenalog, Aristocort
        Hydrocortisone valerate cream 0.2%: Westcort
        Fluocinolone acetonide cream 0.025%: Synalar, Fluonid

    c. Strong corticosteroid preparations
        Amcinonide ointment 0.1%: Cyclocort
        Fluocinonide cream, ointment, gel 0.05%: Lidex
        Halcinonide cream 0.1%: Halog
        Desoximetasone cream 0.25%: Topicort

    d. Very strong corticosteroids
        Clobetasol propionate 0.05% cream and ointment: Demovate
        Betamethasone dipropionate: Diprosone ointment

R.37. Combined preparations containing corticosteroids:

Topical creams and ointments containing corticosteroids in combination with other medications are limited in the United States but are widely used in Europe, especially the combination with antibiotics and/or antimycotics. Such preparations are often unnecessary and could induce the physician to do an inadequate diagnostic workup. Moreover, topical application of aminoglycoside antibiotics (such as gentamicin) is somewhat risky because of the possible development of resistant organisms. Topical neomycin can cause contact allergy, especially with repeated use on damaged skin. The combination of antiseptic agents and corticosteroids may be accepted.

    a. Iodochlorhydroxyquin and hydrocortisone: Vioform hydrocortisone cream, ointment, lotion

The combination of corticosteroids and urea or salicylic acid is useful to improve penetration and effectiveness.

    b. Hydrocortisone-urea: Carmol–HC

    c. Flumetasone (0.02%)/salicylic acid (3%): Locasalen ointment
        Betamethasone (0.1%)/salicylic acid (3%):
            Betnesalic ointment   These preparations
        Fluprednilden (0.1%)/salicylic acid (3%):   must be compounded
            Sali Decoderm ointment   in the United States

Combinations of corticosteroids and tar have anti-inflammatory and antipruritic effects and are useful in chronic eczema. These combinations are not commercially available in the United States.

d. Hydrocortisone (0.4%)/Ichthyol (3%): Ichtho-Cortin ointment
Hydrocortisone (0.2%)/Ichthyol (2%): Ichtho-Cortin cream

R.38. Antiparasitic:

Crotamiton: Eurax cream and lotion
Gamma benzene hexachloride (lindane): Kwell (cream, lotion), Scabene (cream, lotion)
5–10% sulfur ointment (must be compounded)
Benzyl benzoate 20–25% lotion MSP (can be used during pregnancy)

R.39. Antieczematous, antipruritic:

a. Formulations with tar extracts (i.e., 5% liquor carbonis detergens–LCD) or petroleum additives (up to 5% Ichthyol, Tumenol)
b. Ichthyol 10–50% (i.e., Ichtholan 10, 20, 50%) is listed in the German text for enhancing the breakdown of abscess-forming inflammation.
Caution: Coal tars are photosensitizing. They are carcinogenic for the skin of experimental animals, so the risk with long-term therapeutic application must be taken into consideration. With extensive applications, damage to the kidneys is possible.

R.40. Scale-removing:

a. Salicyl-Vaseline
Rx: Salicylic acid 3–5% in white petrolatum. Avoid prolonged total body use. Toxic effect from percutaneous absorption of salicylic acid is possible.
b. Urea ointment
Rx: Urea   10.0
     Aqu. purif.   30.0
     Ungt. Cordes ad 100.0
Commercial preparations:
Aquacare HP (10% urea cream)
Carmol 20 (20% urea) cream
Carmol 10 (10% urea) lotion

R.41. Wound ointments, ulcer medications:

There are a large number of different ointments that often contain more than five individual substances. Conclusive evidence for their effectiveness has been demonstrated for only a few individual components. Also, some of the more frequently used ingredients can cause contact allergies and often do (balsam of Peru, neomycin, benzocaine, sulfonamides). Local factors are more important for wound healing than are topical medications. In poorly healing wounds (leg ulcers, decubitus ulcers, radiation ulcers) treatment of these local factors must take priority (see pp. 19, 25, 129). In the absence of disturbing factors, a simple wound heals under a protective bandage that is permeable to air. Firmly adherent coating on a leg ulcer may occasionally require the use of enzyme preparations:

Santyl ointment (collagenase)
Elase ointment or solution (fibrinolysin and desoxyribonuclease)
Travase (Sutilains)

R.42. Acne medication:

Besides the primarily prescribed gels, creams and the less oily emulsions are also useful, especially for more sensitive skin.

a. Benzoyl peroxide
Clearasil cream
b. Tretinoin, vitamin A acid
Retin A cream

R.43. Sunscreen preparations:

Most of the modern sunscreen preparations contain PABA (para aminobenzoic acid) or its esters or benzophenone derivatives. PABA protects the skin against ultraviolet light (wavelengths 280 to 320 nm). Light of longer wavelengths and visible light penetrates PABA and causes tanning of the skin. PABA alone has a sun protective factor (SPF) of 4 to 10.

Benzophenone derivatives do not provide the same light protection as PABA. They filter a broader spectrum of UV rays, namely the wavelengths between 250 and 400 nm. PABA in combination with benzophenone derivatives provides a protective factor of 10 to 15. Other sunscreen preparations contain zinc oxide or titanium dioxide. They are completely impermeable for visible light and UV radiation, but since they are pastes, they are sometimes cosmetically unsatisfactory.

Some commercially available preparations and their sun protective factor (SPF) are as follows:

> *SPF of 15 or more*
> SolBar Plus 15 cream
> Super Shade 15 (Coppertone) cream
> *SPF between 8 and 14*
> Deleal Sun cream
> Pabafilm 10 gel
> Pabafilm 10 lotion
> PabaGel
> *SPF between 4 and 7*
> Sundown 4 Sunscreen cream
> Sundown 6 Sunscreen cream
> *Complete light protection*
> RV Plaque (RVP + zinc oxide)
> RV Plus (RVP + titanium)
> Solar (PABA + titanium)

I. Corticosteroid-Crystal Suspension

R.44.

Intralesional injection of a corticosteroid-crystal suspension with the Dermojet (principle of the inoculation pistol) or by syringe and needle represents especially intensive forms of local corticosteroid therapy. It is extremely important to avoid injecting the drug into the subcutaneous tissue (long-lasting fat atrophy).

> Triamcinolone: Kenalog or Aristocort
> Betamethasone: Celestone

Medications for Systemic Therapy

The following discussion includes commonly known medications also used for other indications as well as drugs prescribed especially for the treatment of skin diseases.

A. Antibiotics

R.45. Penicillins:
Oral: V-Cillin-K
Pentids
Pen-Vee-K
Parenteral: Bicillin
Wycillin

R.46. Broad-spectrum penicillins:
Amoxicillin, Ampicillin
Amoxicillin plus clavulanate potassium (Augmentin), effective against beta lactamase–forming bacteria

R.47. Tetracyclines:
Tetracycline: Achromycin, Sumycin
Oxytetracycline: Terramycin
Minocycline: Minocin
Doxycycline: Doxycycline, Vibramycin (also available for i.v. injection)

R.48. Oral cefalosporines:
Cefalexin: Keflex
Cephradine: Anspor, Velosef
Cefaclor: Ceclor
Caution: Possible cross allergies with penicillin.

R.49. Erythromycin:
Erythrocin

R.50. Clindamycin:
Clindamycin is a reserve antibiotic for anaerobic infections, not a routine antibiotic for acne therapy.
Cleocin

R.51. Spectinomycin:
Trobicin, exclusively for treatment of gonorrhea

R.52. Rosoxacin:
Winuron for oral treatment of gonorrhea

B. Antimycotics

Systemic therapy is necessary for widespread or markedly inflammatory dermatomycoses that cannot be controlled with topical therapy, especially when the hair is involved. For mycoses of the nails, which require treatment, local therapy is often insufficient. Two medications are presently available for oral therapy:

R.53. Griseofulvin:
The drug is effective selectively against dermatophytes. Undesirable side effects are relatively rare. They include gastrointestinal disturbances, headaches, dizziness, sleeplessness, paresthesias, and very rarely leucopenia.

Griseofulvin (micronized): Grifulvin V; Grisactin

Griseofulvin (ultramicronized): Gris-PE6, Grisactin Ultra, Fulvicin P/G.

These drugs can be given in lower doses, since absorption is better.

R.54. Ketoconazole:
Broad-spectrum antimycotic; effective against dermatophytes and yeasts. Undesirable side effects are rare (nausea, headaches, pruritus, gastrointestinal disturbances). There have been reported disturbances of liver function (some fatal), however, and the drug is no longer recommended for the treatment of onychomycoses.

Nizoral tablets

C. Virustatic Drugs

R.55.
At present, Acyclovir is the most important systemic virustatic drug for dermatologic therapy.

Acyclovir: Zovirax tablets, solution for i.v. therapy.

D. Antihistamines

For dermatologic therapy, we use mainly H-receptor blockers. They are most effective for acute urticaria and hay fever. They are also effective in the treatment of chronic urticaria and other allergic skin reactions. Their effectiveness is limited, however, against pruritus of other etiologies. Here the effect of nonsedating antihistamines is barely more than that of a placebo.

For practical purposes, antihistamines can be divided into those with and those without a sedative component. The component is welcome in the treatment of sleep disturbances caused by pruritus; it is not desirable in a day medication (responsiveness, traffic safety). Combinations of antihistamines with caffeine to reduce the sedative effect or with corticosteroids are not very meaningful because of their dissimilar pharmacokinetics.

R.56. Antihistamine with little or no sedative effect:
Terfenadine: Seldane

Tripelennamine hydrochloride: Pyribenzamine:

R.57. Antihistamines with sedative effect:
Promethazine: Phenergan

Hydroxyzine: Atarax, Durrax

Chlorpheniramine: Chlor-Trimeton

Bamipin: Soventol

Clemastin: Tavist

Cyproheptadine: Periactin

E. Corticosteroids

R.58.

Dermatologic indications for systemic corticosteroid therapy are severe and widespread diseases or acute problems that require a rapid therapeutic effect (drug reactions, diseases of the pemphigus group) as well as skin diseases with concomitant involvement of internal organs, such as lupus erythematosus. Undesirable side effects and contraindications of corticosteroid therapy must be kept in mind, especially in chronic illnesses that require long-term therapy. These problems include Cushing syndrome, hypertension, osteoporosis, a diabetogenic effect, edemata, peptic ulcers, glaucoma, cataracts, immunosuppression with an increased incidence of infections, increased risk of thrombosis, and induction of psychoses. For practical purposes, knowledge of a few selected corticosteroids and their effective strengths is sufficient.

Table II

Drug	Cushing Threshold (mg)	Lowest Dose With Anti-inflammatory Effect (mg)	Commercial Preparations
Hydrocortisone	40	40	Cortef tablets
Prednisone	10	7	Deltasone tablets, Meticor-ten tablets
Prednisolone	10	7	Delta-Cortef tablets
6-Methylprednisolone	8	5	Medrol tablets
Triamcinolone	8	5	Aristocort tablets, Kenacort tablets
Dexamethasone	2	1	Decadron tablets
Betamethasone	2	1	Celestone tablets

For long-term treatment corticosteroids are given according to the circadian rhythm of cortisone secretion: in the morning, or preferably every other morning (alternating administration), provided the status of the disease permits it. Systemic corticosteroid administration with injection of depot preparations does not allow adequate regulation of cortisone; it also causes significant suppression of the adrenal cortex and is not recommended. Combinations of corticosteroids and other active medications, especially antihistamines, are not indicated in dermatologic practice.

Low-dose cortisone therapy as discussed here means administration of the drug in the lowest anti-inflammatory dose, if possible, below the Cushing level (Table II). A median dose would have an equivalent of 30 to 50 mg prednisone; a high dose would be equivalent to 100 mg of prednisone or more per day.

F. Retinoids

Retinoids, derivatives of vitamin A, have become more important in dermatotherapy in recent years. The use of these drugs is still relatively limited because not enough is known about their therapeutic spectrum. Similar medications are still being evaluated. It is possible that these substances will eventually have a therapeutic significance similar to that of corticosteroids.

Undesired side effects include dry lips, loss of hair, and thinning of the skin, especially in the palmar and plantar areas. Elevation of blood fats and of the hepatic enzymes is observed occasionally. These parameters must be checked at regular intervals during treatment with retinoids. Long-term therapy with retinoids can lead to bone changes (hyperostoses), which have been observed mainly in children.

Because of the present state of our knowledge, and to insure economic prescribing of these expensive preparations, it is desirable to consult an experienced dermatologist before prescribing oral synthetic retinoids. At this time, two preparations are available for systemic therapy: Etretinate and Isotretinoin.

R.59. Etretinate (Tegison):

Indications: Severe psoriasis, especially pustular psoriasis, psoriatic erythroderma, and psoriatic arthritis, as well as several hereditary disorders of keratinization and lichen planus. Other possible indications that are still experimental at this time include lupus erythematosus chronicus, progressive scleroderma, cutaneous T-cell lymphoma, and pre-invasive leukoplakia.

The most significant limitation in the therapeutic use of Etretinate is the drug's teratogenic effect. Because of the long half life, one must be certain that the patient does not become pregnant until at least 2 years after discontinuation of the drug.

R.60. Isotretinoin (Accutane):

Indications: Severe forms of acne, especially acne conglobata, severe rosacea.

Since the drug's half life is relatively short compared to Etretinate, conception must be avoided until 4 weeks after discontinuation of the therapy, as well as during the entire course of therapy.

Compression Bandages

Compression bandages are important therapeutic aids in dermatology. Their effectiveness depends a great deal on the technique of application and the materials used.

Compression bandages are prescribed prophylactically to prevent emboli and thromboses, especially in bed-ridden patients. Therapeutically, they are used for treatment of insufficiency of the leg veins or lymphedema. Compression bandages are contraindicated in arterial occlusive disease stages III and IV.

In patients in whom the condition of the skin requires frequent wound care (e.g., leg ulcers, stasis dermatitis), dressings and bandages are changed every day. The following chapter discusses the materials available for these dressings.

Bandages with short tension tracts exert a strong working pressure and have a significant depth effect. They are used for compression therapy in ambulatory patients. Correct application of a compression bandage requires some practice.

Bandages with medium or long tension tracts have a higher resting pressure and are more suitable for the prophylaxis of thromboses in bed-ridden patients. They are more elastic and easier to apply.

Fixed bandages, such as Unna's paste bandages or adhesive bandages, are left in place for several days. They are usually applied by the physician and fit better.

Compression stockings are of benefit for patients in whom no special wound care is necessary and are easier to apply. They should be custom-made and can be obtained as calf-sleeves, below-knee stockings, full-length stockings, and pantyhose, depending on the extent of the venous insufficiency. *Caution*: Calf-sleeves, especially those of the higher compression categories, may cause edema of the foot.

Ready-made support stockings are *not* appropriate for compression therapy.

Compression stockings are available for various indications in the following compression categories:

>*Compression Cagegory I*
>>Ankle pressure 20 mm Hg
>>For mild varicosities (beginning varicosities of pregnancy)
>
>*Compression Category II*
>>Ankle pressure 30 mm Hg
>>For severe varicosities with occasional edema
>
>*Compression Category III*
>>Ankle pressure 40 mm Hg
>>For sequelae of ulcus cruris (leg ulcer), post-thrombotic syndrome
>
>*Compression Category IV*
>>Ankle pressure >60 mm Hg
>>For lymphedema

It must be kept in mind that the material becomes stiffer in the higher compression categories, and more strength is necessary to apply the stockings. This is especially important in older women who may not wear the stockings if they are too hard to put on. Since mild compression is better than no compression at all, it may then be wise to prescribe a pair of stockings with less compression than is actually indicated.

A new pair of stockings must be prescribed every 6 months when continuous compression treatment is necessary and the stockings are worn regularly.

Index

Note: Page numbers in *italics* refer to illustrations.